Tendon Transfers and Treatment Strategies in Foot and Ankle Surgery

Editor

BRUCE E. COHEN

FOOT AND ANKLE CLINICS

www.foot.theclinics.com

Consulting Editor
MARK S. MYERSON

March 2014 • Volume 19 • Number 1

ELSEVIER

1600 John F. Kennedy Boulevard • Suite 1800 • Philadelphia, Pennsylvania, 19103-2899

http://www.theclinics.com

FOOT AND ANKLE CLINICS Volume 19, Number 1
March 2014 ISSN 1083-7515, ISBN-13: 978-0-323-28706-7

Editor: Jennifer Flynn-Briggs

Foot and Ankle Clinics (ISSN 1083-7515) is published quarterly by Elsevier, Inc., 360 Park Avenue South, New York, NY 10010-1710. Months of issue are March, June, September, and December. Periodicals postage paid at New York, NY, and additional mailing offices. Subscription price per year is $315.00 (US individuals), $421.00 (US institutions), $155.00 (US students), $360.00 (Canadian individuals), $506.00 (Canadian institutions), $215.00 (Canadian students), $460.00 (foreign individuals), $506.00 (foreign institutions), and $215.00 (foreign students). To receive student/resident rate, orders must be accompanied by name of affiliated institution, date of term, and the *signature* of program/residency coordinator on institution letterhead. Orders will be billed at individual rate until proof of status is received. Foreign air speed delivery is included in all *Clinics* subscription prices. All prices are subject to change without notice. **POSTMASTER:** Send address changes to *Foot and Ankle Clinics*, Elsevier Health Sciences Division, Subscription Customer Service, 3251 Riverport Lane, Maryland Heights, MO 63043. **Customer Service: 1-800-654-2452 (US and Canada). From outside of the United States and Canada, call 314-447-8871. Fax: 314-447-8029. E-mail: JournalsCustomerService-usa@ elsevier.com (for print support); JournalsOnlineSupport-usa@elsevier.com (for online support).**

Reprints. For copies of 100 or more, of articles in this publication, please contact the Commercial Reprints Department, Elsevier Inc., 360 Park Avenue South, New York, NY 10010-1710. Tel.: 212-633-3874; Fax: 212-633-3820; E-mail: reprints@elsevier.com.

Printed and bound by CPI Group (UK) Ltd, Croydon, CR0 4YY

Contributors

CONSULTING EDITOR

MARK S. MYERSON, MD
Director, The Institute for Foot and Ankle Reconstruction, Mercy Medical Center, Baltimore, Maryland

EDITOR

BRUCE E. COHEN, MD
OrthoCarolina Foot and Ankle Institute, Charlotte, North Carolina

AUTHORS

MOSTAFA ABOUSAYED, MD
Department of Orthopaedics, Massachusetts General Hospital, Orthopaedic Associates, Boston, Massachusetts

JONATHON D. BACKUS, MD
Resident, Department of Orthopaedic Surgery, Washington University School of Medicine in St Louis, St Louis, Missouri

ERIC M. BLUMAN, MD, PhD
Assistant Professor of Orthopedic Surgery, Harvard Medical School, Boston, Massachusetts

THOMAS DOWD, MD
Chief, Foot and Ankle Service, Department of Orthopaedics and Rehabilitation, San Antonio Military Medical Center, Fort Sam, Houston, Texas

DANIEL C. FARBER, MD
Chief, Foot and Ankle Service, University of Maryland Medical Center, Assistant Professor, Department of Orthopaedics University of Maryland School of Medicine, Chief, University of Maryland Orthopaedics and Rehabilitation Institute, Baltimore, Maryland; Assistant Professor of Clinical Orthopaedic Surgery, University of Pennsylvania, Philadelphia, Pennsylvania

KENNETH J. HUNT, MD
Assistant Professor, Department of Orthopaedics, Stanford University, Redwood City, California

TODD A. IRWIN, MD
Assistant Professor, Department of Orthopaedic Surgery, University of Michigan Hospital System, Ann Arbor, Michigan

CARROLL P. JONES, MD
OrthoCarolina, Charlotte, North Carolina

GEORGIOS C. KARAOGLANIS, MD
Attending Orthopaedic Surgeon, Orthopaedic Department, 401 General Army Hospital, Athens, Greece

BRANDON W. KING, MD
Resident, Department of Orthopaedic Surgery, University of Michigan Hospital System, Ann Arbor, Michigan

JOHN Y. KWON, MD
Department of Orthopaedics, Massachusetts General Hospital, Orthopaedic Associates, Boston, Massachusetts

EDWARD LANSANG, MD, FRCSC
University Health Network- Toronto Western Division, Western Hospital, Toronto, Ontario, Canada

JOHNNY LAU, MD, MSc, FRCSC
Assistant Professor, University of Toronto, Consultant, University Health Network, Toronto, Ontario, Canada

JEREMY J. MCCORMICK, MD
Assistant Professor in Foot and Ankle Surgery, Department of Orthopaedic Surgery, Washington University School of Medicine in St Louis, Chesterfield, Missouri

STEVEN K. NEUFELD, MD
Medical Director, Orthopaedic Foot and Ankle Center of Washington, Falls Church; Clinical Professor, Department of Orthopaedic Surgery, Virginia Commonwealth University, Richmond, Virginia

CRISTIAN ORTIZ, MD
Orthopedic Department, Clinica Alemana, Vitacura, Santiago, Chile

VINOD KUMAR PANCHBHAVI, MD, FACS
Chief, Division of Foot & Ankle Surgery, Director of Foot & Ankle Fellowship Program, Professor, Department of Orthopedic Surgery, University of Texas Medical Branch, Galveston, Texas

DAVID J. RUTA, MD
Resident, Department of Orthopaedic Surgery, University of Michigan Hospital System, Ann Arbor, Michigan

JESSICA H. RYU, MD
Orthopaedic Resident, Department of Orthopaedics, Stanford University, Redwood City, California

KARL M. SCHWEITZER Jr, MD
OrthoCarolina, Charlotte, North Carolina

EMMANOUIL D. STAMATIS, Lt Colonel, MD, FHCOS, FACS, PhD
Attending Orthopaedic Surgeon, Orthopaedic Department, 401 General Army Hospital, Athens, Greece

ANDREA VELJKOVIC, MD, FRCSC
Foot and Ankle Reconstruction/Arthroscopy & Athletic Injuries, Lecturer, Division of Orthopaedics, Department of Surgery, University of Toronto; University Health Network-Toronto Western Division, Toronto, Ontario, Canada

EMILIO WAGNER, MD
Orthopedic Department, Clinica Alemana, Vitacura, Santiago, Chile

Contents

depending on the muscle deficiency and the function to restore, different tendon transfer options exist. The authors do not recommend tendon transfers for forefoot deformities in this setting. Postoperatively tendon transfers should be protected in a removable boot, but early protected weight bearing and motion is stimulated to obtain a well-functioning transfer and not a tenodesis.

FOOT AND ANKLE CLINICS

Preface

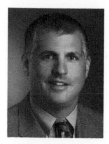

Bruce E. Cohen, MD
Editor

I am very pleased to serve as the guest editor for this issue of *Foot and Ankle Clinics of North America*. We have a great lineup of authors who have done a fantastic job covering our topic: Tendon Transfers and Treatment Strategies in Foot and Ankle Surgery.

Tendon transfers have always interested me due to the complexity and variability of the deformities. An understanding of the pathologic condition and deforming forces is critical to adequately utilize these types of treatments effectively. Effective and successful surgical reconstruction involves more than just performing an osseous reconstruction or tendon release, it involves moving a musculotendon unit in an effective manner to correct a deformity.

To begin the discussion of the use of these powerful procedures, we must first understand how to evaluate a neuromuscular deformity and how a tendon transfer works. These topics are covered in our first two articles.

Specific pathologic conditions are the topics for the remaining articles, where the use of tendon transfers is highlighted. The specific topics/conditions covered include flatfoot, cavovarus deformities, hallux and lesser toe deformities, foot drop, Achilles dysfunction, peroneal reconstruction, and the spastic foot. In addition, Vinod Panchbhavi, MD presents some cutting-edge percutaneous techniques for various tendon transfers.

I would personally like to thank all of my authors for their contributions. We need to acknowledge the hard work and expertise it requires to create these fine articles. Finally, I would like to thank Mark Myerson and the editorial staff at Elsevier for their assistance with this issue. This periodical continues be a superior publication that provides an outstanding forum for presentation of foot and ankle topics and techniques. *Foot and Ankle Clinics of North America* is still a "go-to" resource for current up-to-date coverage of important topics in our field.

I hope you enjoy this issue and, even more, I hope you begin or continue to use these techniques in your practice.

Bruce E. Cohen, MD
OrthoCarolina Foot and Ankle Institute
2001 Vail Avenue, Suite 200B
Charlotte, NC 28207, USA

E-mail address:
Bruce.Cohen@OrthoCarolina.com

Foot Ankle Clin N Am 19 (2014) ix
http://dx.doi.org/10.1016/j.fcl.2013.12.001
1083-7515/14/$ – see front matter © 2014 Elsevier Inc. All rights reserved.

Neuromuscular Problems in Foot and Ankle: Evaluation and Workup

Kenneth J. Hunt, MD*, Jessica H. Ryu, MD

KEYWORDS

- Neuromuscular foot • Charcot-Marie-Tooth • Clubfoot • Muscular dystrophy
- Cerebral palsy • Spina bifida • Myelomeningocele

KEY POINTS

- Neuromuscular disorders of the foot and ankle are important to recognize, understand, and accurately diagnose. It is essential to determine the functional goals of the patient during the workup and particularly treatment planning stages.
- Accurate diagnosis, and informed discussion of treatment options. Must be in the context of the patient's disease, cognition, comorbidities, functional attributes, and family environment.
- Regardless of cause, a thorough history and physical examination aid in an appropriate diagnostic workup and optimal orthopedic management of each patient.

INTRODUCTION

Neuromuscular disorders include a spectrum of conditions that affect the spinal cord, peripheral nerves, neuromuscular junctions, and muscles. Both congenital and acquired neurologic conditions can profoundly affect the shape and function of the foot, ankle, and lower extremities. To optimize the orthopedic management of these patients, it is vital to identify and accurately diagnose the underlying cause of foot and ankle deformity or disability. Accurate diagnosis is important in defining prognosis, likelihood of progression, selection of appropriate treatment modalities, and patient/family counseling.

The diagnosis is often made from clinical history, detailed family history, and physical examination. However, for the various disorders, several adjunctive tests can be vital to the diagnosis, including:

- Laboratory tests (eg, serum enzyme studies, creatine kinase, and aldolase)
- Genetic testing

Disclosures: Neither author has any financial relationships that would produce a conflict of interest.

Department of Orthopaedics, Stanford University, 450 Broadway Street, MC 6342, Redwood City, CA 94063, USA

* Corresponding author.

E-mail address: kjhunt@stanford.edu

- Electromyography (EMG) and nerve conduction velocity studies
- Nerve and muscle biopsies

This article focuses on evaluation and workup for common congenital and acquired neuromuscular conditions that affect the foot and ankle. Some general principles of the diagnostic process are explored, followed by discussion of specific congenital and acquired disorders commonly encountered by orthopedic foot and ankle specialists.

GENERAL HISTORY AND PHYSICAL EXAMINATION

Neurologic abnormalities can manifest with an imbalance of available muscular function. It is important that all individuals with suspected neurologic conditions be carefully assessed in the context of their disease. History should include onset, timing, frequency, and severity of symptoms and the resulting functional limitations. Parents and caregivers can be important providers of information, depending on the patient's age and cognitive function. Evaluation of feet, ankles, and lower extremities is important for an adequate physical examination, but the examiner must be prepared to assess the entire neurologic and musculoskeletal system. A precise diagnosis can often be reached through careful history, a thorough physical examination, and by use of select specific laboratory and imaging procedures.

The examination technique of the foot and ankle can vary based on patient age. For example, in examination of an infant, inspection, palpation, and manipulation must be relied on, whereas in the older child and adults, these techniques can be supplemented with observations of ambulation and other activities.[1] The examiner should consider the foot and ankle as parts of the entire body and an important part of the locomotion system. They should not be considered static in nature, because they are subject to anatomic and functional variation during activities.

Strength testing to detect symmetric or asymmetric muscle weakness is an important part of the clinical evaluation. Strength can be assessed by observing activities such as walking and dressing and by testing individual muscle groups. Evaluation of muscle strength can help localize the distribution of weakness. Be aware of associated fixed deformities, because these may affect the examination.[2] Both agonist and antagonist muscles are graded for strength throughout range of motion and in all planes.

Deep tendon reflexes of the patella and Achilles should be tested. The quality of the reflex is assessed by the briskness of muscle contracture and should be graded as absent, hypoactive, normal, or hyperactive. Clonus is generally a description used for reflexes as well. For example, children with muscular dystrophy have normal reflexes until later in the course of the disease, after which they become weaker.[3,4] Also important in workup of neuromuscular disorders is sensory status. In neuropathies, there can be a glove or stocking distribution of loss, paresthesias, pins and needles sensation, and even dysesthesia.

ASSESSMENT OF GAIT

Observation of the patient's gait is a useful component of the physical examination, particularly of a child. The examiner should review at least 6 stride pairs in both the anteroposterior (AP) and lateral direction during each walk. The examiner should watch the patient's foot placement, and whether this is a heel-toe disposition with a triple rocker, flat-footed placement with inversion or eversion, toe-heel placemen, or persistent dynamic equinus. These entities represent degrees of increasing severity of the hemiplegic gait. The normal process of ambulation involves progression of the hip flexors on 1 side, then heel strike and weight bearing. As the individual shifts their weight onto the contralateral hip, the contralateral leg begins heel rise and eventual toe off. The clinician's ability to identify these different gait patterns can allow the clinician to distinguish abnormal gaits, such as the congenital or acquired hemiplegic gait, the diplegic gait, the gait of Duchenne, peripheral neuropathy, and so forth.

MUSCLE AND NERVE BIOPSY

When indicated, a biopsy of muscle or nerve can be valuable for the definitive diagnosis of a neuromuscular disorder. The biopsy should be taken from a muscle that is involved but is still functioning (usually the gastrocnemius or vastus lateralis). Muscles with mild involvement should be selected in chronic disease, and severely involved muscle should be chosen in acute disease. Atraumatic technique is essential to preserve architecture. A muscle biopsy specimen should be about 10 mm long and 3 mm deep and should be fixed in glutaraldehyde (for electron microscopy) or liquid nitrogen (for light microscopy). The specimen should not be placed into saline solution or formalin. For nerve biopsy, when necessary, the sural nerve is usually chosen. This nerve can be accessed at the posterolateral ankle between the Achilles tendon and the lateral malleolus just proximal to the level of the tibiotalar joint. The entire width of the nerve should be taken for a length of 3 to 4 cm.

NEUROMUSCULAR ULTRASONOGRAPHY

Another useful parameter to consider while assessing muscle may be ultrasonographic echogenicity. Healthy muscle tissue is normally dark and echolucent on ultrasonography. However, in myopathies and neurogenic disorders, muscle tissue undergoes atrophy, necrosis, inflammation, and fibrosis; because of this situation, diseased muscle is more echogenic, and there is loss of normal tissue heterogeneity and its surrounding fibrous stroma.[5] Among the benefits of muscle ultrasonography is that it can be been used to track changes in muscle size in progressive neuromuscular disorders. Studies have shown that patients with childhood motor neuron disease and muscular dystrophy with longer duration or severity of symptoms have smaller muscle size on ultrasonography. For example, the pseudohypertrophy of muscles in Duchenne muscular dystrophy is a finding that ultrasonography can readily quantify.[5]

GENETIC EVALUATION

Significant advances have been made in our knowledge of the genetic basis of neuromuscular disorders. Through innovations in molecular biology, chromosome locations for various abnormal genes have been identified, characterized, and sequenced. In addition to genetic sequencing, we now understand the biochemical basis for some diseases. For example, the region for the gene responsible for Duchenne and Becker muscular dystrophy provides coding for the dystrophin protein. Testing for dystrophin can be used as a biochemical test for muscular dystrophy and to differentiate Duchenne muscular dystrophy from Becker muscular dystrophy. Patients suspected of a disorder with a genetic basis should be appropriately referred for genetic testing.

DIAGNOSTIC APPROACH TO NEUROMUSCULAR DISORDERS

For the purposes of this article, specific disorders are separated into congenital and acquired. A brief description of what is known about the disorder is followed by guidelines for evaluation and workup for each disorder.

Congenital Neurologic Disorders

Hereditary motor sensory neuropathy

There are many clinically and genetically distinct diseases in which abnormalities of sensory motor nerves are the root cause of the condition. These conditions must be distinguished from those in which peripheral neuropathy is part of a more generalized neuraxial abnormality, such as Friedreich ataxia, and from sensory neuropathies, in which the motor nerves are unaffected but may result in neuropathic joints, ulceration, and fractures. The most common hereditary motor sensory neuropathy (HMNS), Charcot-Marie-Tooth (CMT), is a complicated group of more than 50 inherited, progressive peripheral neuropathies. They are hypothesized to result from an abnormality of myelination. CMT is the most common inherited disorder of the peripheral nerves, affecting approximately 36 people out of every 100,000.[6]

Type I HMSN is the classic and most common presentation of CMT disease. This autosomal-dominant disease is characterized by slow nerve conduction velocities, usually presenting in the second decade of life.[7] The measurement of nerve conduction velocities is the most important primary tool for diagnosis.[6] Most type I presentations have been linked to chromosome 17 and are designated CMT 1A.[8]

Type II HMSN has a similar presentation but is less severe and usually appears later in life. In type II, the rate of impulse transfer is normal, but the magnitude of impulse is decreased. Nerve conductions are seldom slower, and if so, they are only mildly decreased.[9] In general, CMT affects the longest nerves to the smallest muscles first. The most common lower extremity presentation is bilateral pes cavovarus deformities with leg weakness,[10] but there can also be progressive weakness of the upper extremities occurring later in the disease course. Hip dysplasia and scoliosis can also be present.[11]

Workup A comprehensive neurologic evaluation is necessary when CMT is suspected. If the patient presents in early childhood, a slightly valgus foot with shortened calf muscles may be the only finding noted on physical examination. In subsequent years, patients with CMT develop a pes cavovarus deformity, combined with decreased proprioception, resulting in a motor imbalance between pairs of muscles around the foot and ankle.[12] A recent study[6] showed that 78% of children with bilateral cavovarus deformity have CMT. Children who have late dysplasia and a broad-based gait should undergo a CMT evaluation.[13] The most common examination finding includes significant weakness of the tibialis anterior and peroneus brevis muscles.[14,15] The functioning peroneus longus results in plantarflexion of the first ray, a cavus foot, and a compensatory hindfoot varus (**Fig. 1**). The hindfoot varus is exacerbated by the unopposed pull of the tibialis posterior.

Another common deformity in CMT is clawing of the toes (see **Fig. 1**). The extensor hallucis longus and extensor digitorum longus are recruited to dorsiflex the ankle, resulting in loading imbalance and toe clawing.[14,16] The claw deformity is caused by intrinsic muscle weakness that allows the long toe flexor muscles to flex the interphalangeal joint and the long toe extensor muscles to extend the metatarsophalangeal joint.

Gait examination shows a characteristic steppage gait stemming from the combination of dorsiflexion weakness, fixed equines, and difficulties with proprioception. The hindfoot is noted to be in equinus with limited dorsiflexion, and there is often hyperextension of the knee and overload of the lateral border of the foot. During the swing phase, a foot drop and foot clearance issues are noted as a result of tibialis anterior weakness.

During workup of suspected CMT, there is a sensory neuropathy component as well. Early changes can be subtle, primarily with loss of proprioceptive and vibratory

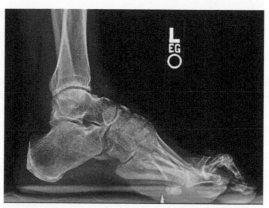

Fig. 1. Lateral radiograph of patient with CMT disease. Note the presence of a plantarflexed first ray, increased calcaneal pitch angle, and claw toe deformities.

sense. Sensory presentations can vary greatly, and patients are less inclined to recognize or acknowledge the diminished sensation, but this deficit can limit their ability to balance properly. Up to 25% of patients have a significant sensory impairment, and vibration, 2-point discrimination, and proprioception are the first to be affected.[17] The common peroneal nerve is one of the early nerves to be affected. In addition to sensory loss, the decreased proprioception results in difficulty ambulating, lack of balance, and painful calluses.[18] As the foot deformity becomes more severe and fixed, painful calluses can develop over the heel, lateral foot, and first metatarsal head.[18] Also, it is not uncommon to have early loss of the Achilles tendon reflex, although the patellar reflux survives for longer.[6]

The Coleman block test (Fig. 2) is a fundamental tool of the assessment of cavovarus foot deformity.[19] This test is performed by allowing the plantarflexed first metatarsal to hang over a 2.5-cm block, which eliminates the forced forefoot pronation; if the heel returns to a neutral position, the hindfoot deformity is flexible, and the midfoot and forefoot should be addressed.[4] If the hindfoot does not correct, it is a fixed deformity and the hindfoot must be addressed. The Silfverskiöld test should also be performed to distinguish between isolated gastrocnemius contracture and combined shortening of the gastrocnemius-soleus complex.[6] In this test, the examiner dorsiflexes the ankle with the knee extended and then with the knee bent. If the ankle is

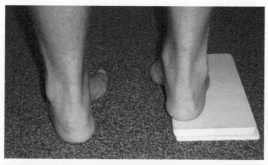

Fig. 2. Coleman block test. The first ray is allowed to drop and hindfoot correction/flexibility is assessed.

unable to passively dorsiflex past neutral, the patient has equinus, and if that motion increases to greater than 10° with the knee flexed, the patient has a gastrocnemius equinus. If there is no change in motion comparing the 2, then it is a combined gastrocnemius-soleus equinus.

Radiographic workup Three standing views of the foot and a hindfoot alignment view should be obtained to assess the ankle joint, hindfoot, calcaneal pitch, and midfoot and forefoot position, and for arthritic changes. The standing lateral radiograph also allows the clinician to estimate the contribution of the hindfoot, midfoot, and forefoot to the cavus deformity (see **Fig. 1**). The AP foot view can help assess for metatarsus adductus. Dynamic pedobarography can be useful to measure the pressure distribution pattern during gait and to identify the primary pressure points and distribution.[6] Magnetic resonance imaging (MRI) shows fatty infiltration in the peroneus brevis and tibialis anterior.[20]

Laboratory workup Although the diagnosis of CMT is often based on history, physical examination, and neurologic assessment, diagnostic tests can be confirmatory.[6] EMG and nerve conduction studies show decreased velocity of nerve impulse conduction and increased charging time.[6] DNA testing is an important part of the workup but is beyond the scope of this discussion. Biopsy of the sural nerve is the ultimate diagnostic test, and presence of well-formed onion bulbs made up of Schwann cell extensions is the typical finding.

Spina bifida and myelomeningocele
Spina bifida is a congenital disorder caused by the incomplete closing of the embryonic neural tube, in which some vertebrae remain unfused and open. A sufficiently large opening may allow a portion of the spinal cord to protrude. Spina bifida malformations fall into 3 categories: spina bifida occulta, spina bifida cystica with meningocele, and spina bifida cystica with myelomeningocele. Myelomeningocele is the most significant and common form, leading to a functional disability in most afflicted individuals.

Patients generally develop significant dwarfing of the lower limbs and short stature, particularly in higher level lesions.[4] Patients with myelomeningocele can be classified into 4 groups based on level of involvement: thoracic, upper lumbar, lower lumbar, and sacral. The thoracic and upper lumbar patients are paralyzed below the knee but might have involuntary motor affecting foot position. The pattern of sensory and motor loss is often asymmetric, and both lower motor neuron and upper motor neuron abnormalities must be considered.

Workup Up to half of children with myelomeningocele have a significant foot deformity. The most common congenital foot deformity is talipes equinovarus or clubfoot deformity (**Fig. 3**).[21] This deformity is generally seen in myelomeningocele of the third lumbar vertebra or above. At this level, the foot is essentially completely paralyzed and insensate. Because of high variability in deficits affecting these patients, and different functional capacities, the treatment must be approached carefully and individually. It is important that the functional motor level be determined, because this determines ambulatory capacity. An important long-term factor is the presence or absence of foot sensation.[22] Patients with the lower lumbar and sacral levels may have partial preservation of plantar foot sensation.

Common foot deformities in myelomeningocele include clubfoot, calcaneovalgus deformity, metatarsus adductus, and congenital vertical talus (CVT). The level of the lesion does not always predict foot deformity, suggesting that the cause is

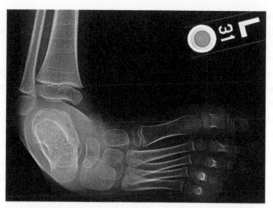

Fig. 3. AP ankle radiograph showing severe equinovarus deformity.

multifactorial.[23] Equinus deformity can occur, and is primarily seen in the completely paralyzed foot and ankle. A calcaneus position foot is common in myelomeningocele, because of the early innervation of foot dorsiflexors in the lower lumbar spine and the late innervation of the gastrocnemius-soleus complex at the sacral levels. Clinically, this deformity results in a relatively plantigrade foot, with no resistance to dorsiflexion of the forefoot, or a dorsiflexed foot, with all weight bearing on the heel, or a calcaneocavus deformity (**Fig. 4**). The calcaneal cavus deformity is usually seen in sacral-level patients with paralysis of the triceps surae, peroneals, and intrinsics. This deformity results in increased plantar pressure beneath the heel and metatarsal heads, and sensation is usually absent along the lateral border of the foot, making recurrent ulcerations a problem. In addition, difficulties with footwear can result from midtarsal bossing and claw toe deformities.

Physical examination Evaluation of the infant or young child with this disorder can be problematic, because it is difficult to assess voluntary or involuntary motor function around the foot and ankle. Because a clubfoot deformity associated with myelomeningocele generally involves the third lumbar level or above, the foot lacks both motor

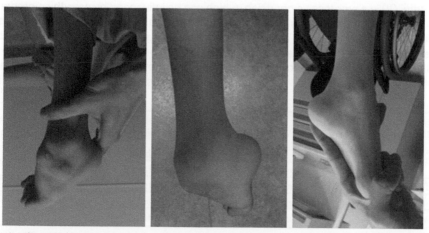

Fig. 4. Clinical photographs of a patient with a history of spina bifida and a 1-year history of acquired equinovarus foot deformity.

function and sensation. Repeat examinations are helpful, as is family input, but hip flexion can sometimes be mistaken for foot motion by the patient's caregivers. The difficulty with motor function assessment is evident in the patient whose unrecognized posterior tibial function results in progressive clubfoot deformity on examination.

In children, careful assessment should be made of the skin or soft tissue dimpling, because those are features of a syndromic foot and are associated with a poor response to treatment. The flexibility of the foot is important, and fixed deformities at each level should be identified and quantified, because this can aid in understanding which structures are limiting joint movement. There are 2 commonly used classification systems, Diméglio[24] and Pirani,[25] and they both apply a point score to various physical findings, which, when summated, differentiate between mildly affected feet that require little or no treatment and the more severely affected foot, which is likely to require treatment (**Table 1**).

Radiographic workup Standard radiographs are difficult to obtain, but may be useful to exclude any obvious bony abnormality, such as a tibial dysplasia, which can be confused as a clubfoot deformity. The lateral and AP talocalcaneal angles should diverge in the normal foot, and if there is parallelism in 1 or both views, this suggests presence of a clubfoot deformity.[26] Computed tomography and MRI can help define the pathoanatomy of the deformity but are not usually used for primary assessment of the clubfoot in the infant.

Cerebral palsy

Cerebral palsy (CP) is a group of developmental disorders that cause abnormal movement and posture, which result in activity restriction or disability.[13] It is believed to be caused by disturbances of the fetal or infant brain. This spectrum of disorders occurs in approximately 0.25% of all live births, and in most cases, a cause cannot be identified.[27] In a multicenter study, Nelson and Ellenberg[28] found that only 21% of children who developed CP had any sign of intrapartum asphyxia and only 9% had asphyxia in the absence of congenital malformation. Maternal mental retardation, low birth weight, and fetal malformation were found to be the leading predictors. All children with CP have some damage to the brain and often have associated disabilities, such as epilepsy, mental handicap, speech disorders, and behavioral disturbances.[27]

Although neurologic damage may not progress, with respect to the musculoskeletal system, CP is a progressive condition, which can be influenced by growth or intervention.[27] Often, the condition is not evident at birth but manifests later as developmental delay. If these children have not begun sitting by the age of 2 years or ambulating by the age of 6 years, they usually do not develop that specific ability later in life.

In CP, there is an incidence of short stature and growth failure, and the limbs are noted to be short and thin. Classification can be based on anatomic (hemiplegia,

Table 1			
The Diméglio system for the classification of congenital equinovarus			
Classification Grade	Type	Score	Reducibility (%)
I	Benign	<5	>90 soft-soft, resolving
II	Moderate	5 to <10	>50 soft-stiff, reducible, partly resistant
III	Severe	10 to <15	<50 stiff-soft, resistant, partly reducible
IV	Very severe	15 to <20	<10 stiff-stiff, resistant

From van Mulken JM, Bulstra SK, Hoefnagels NH. Evaluation of the treatment of clubfeet with the Diméglio score. J Pediatr Orthop 2001;21(5):642–7; with permission.

diplegia, or total body involvement), or physiologic (spastic, athetoid, ataxic, rigid, or mixed) involvement. This classification is often difficult, because there is inaccuracy quantifying the degree of spasticity, athetosis, or ataxia.[27] Children often fit into typical patterns, but there can be overlap. Because of lack of inhibition caused by neurologic injury, spasticity is the primary problem in these patients. In addition, a few of these patients have a movement disorder, which makes evaluation of the foot and ankle deformities more difficult.

Workup Two basic types of foot and ankle deformities are seen in the CP population:

- Varus or equinovarus deformity is noted in the hemiplegic patient
- Equinovalgus deformity is seen more often in the spastic diplegic patient

In the evaluation of both foot and ankle in patients with CP, it is important to determine the functional goals and needs of the patient. Deformity of the foot and ankle is generally not the reason that children with CP do not ambulate.[22,29]

In categorizing function, the Gross Motor Function Classification Scale categorizes patients based on level of ability[13]:

- Level I and II patients are independent ambulators
- Level III patients are dependent ambulators
- Level IV patients can walk very short distances but use a wheelchair for community mobility
- Level V patients are completely nonambulatory, and usually have the lowest level of functioning and the highest disease burden

Physical examination Before gait is observed in the ambulatory child with CP, the patient is seated at the edge of the examination table, allowing the legs to hang freely so the examiner can observe the range of motion of the lower extremity joints without having to move the patient. Stance and gait should be observed next, and coordination and balance can be determined by asking the child to stand or jump on 1 leg.[27] Evaluation of gait is difficult in these patients, because there are usually abnormalities of the trunk, pelvis, hip, knee, ankle, and foot in multiple different planes. A truly comprehensive gait evaluation in a patient with CP includes kinematics, kinetics, energy consumption, and dynamic EMG. Most ambulatory patterns in CP represent the most efficient method of progression, and it may be a compensation for deficient control of equilibrium, joint contracture, or muscle spasticity.[27]

The common pattern for children with CP with hemiplegia or diplegia is internal rotation, flexion, and adduction of the hip. There may also be flexion of the knee and an equinus posture of the ankle.[27] With respect to the foot, a valgus calcaneus and pes valgus are common associated deformities. The foot is commonly affected, and most patients have a mobile hindfoot. The ankle should not be evaluated in isolation because equinus is primarily caused by the contracture of the gastrocnemius or the soleus or secondary to hip or knee flexion contractures. This compensatory equinus position may be used to allow the foot to contact the ground. The 3 common causes of the varus deformity are:

- Spasticity of the tibialis posterior
- Spasticity of the tibialis anterior
- Spasticity of the gastrocnemius-soleus complex

The tibialis posterior spasticity causes hindfoot varus and the tibialis anterior causes midfoot varus (this is the most common deforming force). Rarely, the primary deforming force is the anterior tibialis muscle.

The range of ankle dorsiflexion is measured with the heel held in inversion, stabilizing the talonavicular joint, preventing lateral bow-stringing of the Achilles tendon, and preventing dorsiflexion of the midtarsal joints. If the deformity is varus, the heel must be corrected to a neutral or valgus position. The Silfverskiöld test can differentiate between contractures of the gastrocnemius and the soleus. The amount of ankle dorsiflexion allowed when the foot is released from inversion represents the overall mobility and instability of the hindfoot and midfoot joints. Subtalar and midtarsal movements can then be assessed along with the toes.[27]

Duchenne muscular dystrophy

The muscular dystrophies are a group of inherited muscle disorders characterized by progressive muscle weakness caused by primary degeneration of muscle fibers. Duchenne muscular dystrophy is a sex-linked disorder with clinical onset between 3 and 6 years of age. It is caused by mutation of deletion of DNA at a locus Xp21 on the short arm of the X chromosome, and it occurs in approximately 3 out of 100,000 boys, and can lead to the loss of ambulatory ability and death.[2] The absence of dystrophin and dystrophin-associated glycoproteins results in accumulation of fat in the muscles and fibrous tissues.[2] The child might have slight developmental delay, could be a toe walker, or might have difficulty running or jumping. Pseudohypertrophy of the calf muscles is a common finding, along with the deltoid and serratus anterior. This weakness can result in a wide-based waddling gait with associated increased lumbar lordosis. The clinical progress of Duchenne muscular dystrophy can be followed by a scale to monitor the rate of progression of this degenerating condition, and the different levels are as follows:

1. Walks and climbs stairs without assistance
2. Walks and climbs stairs with aid of railing
3. Walks and climbs stairs slowly with aid of railing
4. Walks unassisted and rises from chair but cannot climb stairs
5. Walks unassisted but cannot rise from chair or climb stairs
6. Walks only with assistance or walks independently with long leg braces
7. Walks in leg braces but requires assistance for balance
8. Stands in long leg braces but unable to walk even with assistance
9. Remains in wheelchair or bed

Slowing of this disease can be achieved clinically by maintaining the child's ability to ambulate, corrective scoliosis surgery, continuous positive airway pressure ventilation, and corticosteroid therapy.[30]

Workup The diagnosis can often be made based on family history, clinical presentation, and an increased serum creatine phosphokinase level. Traditionally, muscle biopsy has been used to confirm the presence of the disease, but DNA analysis using peripheral blood can help to identify carriers and allow for prenatal diagnosis in 70% to 80% of children. Orthopedic treatment is aimed at maintenance of strength and walking ability, and also the prevention of deformities. The most important factor in maintaining strength is prevention of prolonged immobilization.[13] Toe walking, caused by contractures of the Achilles tendon, can be seen in patients as young as 3 years of age.

When discussing the child with the parent, often a history is given of difficulty climbing stairs, hopping, or jumping.[13] On physical examination, boys usually present between the ages of 3 and 6 years, with the chief complaint of delayed walking or toe walking. On physical examination, the clinical features include an enlarged calf and the presence of the traditional physical examination sign, the Gower sign, which is the inability of the patient to rise from the floor without assistance of the upper extremities. Patients can also present with the Trendelenburg sign, and often on examination, proximal muscle weakness is greater than the weakness in the distal musculature. Lumbar lordosis is a common way to compensate for weak gluteal muscles, and circumduction of the limb compensates for weakness of the hip flexors.

CVT

This deformity is also referred to as convex pes valgus, or rocker-bottom foot deformity.[2] It is characterized by a severe hindfoot equinus, a vertical talus with the calcaneus in equinus and valgus (dorsiflexed and everted). The midfoot at the level of the talonavicular and calcaneocuboid joints is dislocated dorsally and cannot be corrected into a neutral position. As with other deformities, isolated muscle function, spasticity, and the patient's functional level may contribute to the degree of deformity. In approximately 50% of cases, CVT is associated with a genetic or neuromuscular disorder.

Workup On examination, the forefoot appears to be dorsiflexed abducted and everted. The pathoanatomy is believed to be a contracture of the evertors and the dorsiflexors.[31] The anterior tibial and peroneus brevis muscles are usually weakened early in the course of the disease. Because of unopposed posterior tibial muscle function, equinus contractures occur initially at the ankle, followed by equinovarus contractures. On radiographic imaging, the lateral plantar flexion radiograph is used to differentiate this condition from oblique talus. In patients with CVT, the talus remains dislocated on this view, whereas in patients with oblique talus, it reduces on a plantar flexion radiograph. On the AP view, a talocalcaneal angle of greater than 40° is consistent with CVT, where normal ranges between 20° and 40° and less than 20° is consistent with clubfoot.

Acquired Neurologic Disorders

The common component of acquired neurologic disorders is that they occur only in the skeletally mature patient, and therefore do not have the impact on bone and joint development that congenital disorders have. Because acquired conditions do not have the same detrimental effects on formation of the foot and ankle, prevention of anticipated or early deformity can be effective.[2] This group of disorders primarily involves the central nervous system and includes cerebrovascular accident (CVA), traumatic brain injury (TBI), and spinal cord injury. Spasticity is usually the primary concern, but as with the congenital neurologic disorders, defining a clear functional goal with respect to treatment of the individual patient is critical.

CVA

On the most basic level, a CVA or stroke is an event in which a blood vessel is obstructed by a clot (embolic) or is affected by a bleed (hemorrhagic), which, in turn, leads to interruption of flow to a portion of the brain. It is the leading cause of adult hemiplegia, and most survivors are able to lead functional lives.[32,33] Each year, about 700,000 people experience a new or recurrent stroke; most (87%) are ischemic, whereas 13% result from intracerebral or subarachnoid hemorrhage.[34] Most patients with stroke develop significant foot and ankle deformity and instability of the lower limb, necessitating orthopedic intervention.

Patients with stroke are at a high risk for falls as a result of many intrinsic physical factors, such as postural imbalance, muscular weakness, and improper flexibility. Most falls occur during activities in which the person is changing positions.[35] The first

6 months after the event are often the most important with respect to regaining function. Patient age, comorbid illnesses, and cause of CVA all influence the extent of and time required to achieve recovery. The degree of gait impairment can vary, but most individuals have decreased walking speed and abnormal gait kinematics after stroke.[35]

The most common foot deformity after stroke in the adult hemiplegic patient is equinovarus. This is a spastic varus deformity of the hindfoot and forefoot, equinus of the ankle and midfoot, and toe flexion. The primary deforming force is the anterior tibialis muscle. This force causes supination of the hindfoot and midfoot into a varus position and contracture of the triceps muscles, resulting in equinovarus posture. All of these factors effectively lengthen the limb, which makes ambulation difficult because of impaired balance and muscle control. Along with this deformity, the posterior tibialis may not function correctly, and there may be spasticity in the flexor hallucis longus, flexor digitorum longus, and the intrinsic musculature of the foot.

Workup Sensory and motor assessment is important in this patient population. With respect to sensory deficits, loss of body awareness is characteristic of a stroke in the parietal region, and often does not allow the patient to ambulate at a functional level. Motor assessment involves the evaluation of strength and the presence or absence of clonus and normal reflexes. The ability of the patient to balance, flex their hip, and remain in a stable position is important for ambulation. Because of the disruption of the upper motor neuron inhibitory pathways after a stroke, muscle spasticity often results. The pattern of spasticity noted in the patient is related to the anatomic region affected. The middle cerebral artery is most often affected, resulting clinically in hemiplegia and greater spasticity in the upper limbs and face compared with the lower extremities. Significant spasticity leading to contracture can involve all of the soft tissues, and also result in the alteration of cartilage and intra-articular fibrosis as a result of long-term immobilization.[2] Clinical evaluation of these patients at an early point involves maintaining range of motion and splinting the patient in a neutral or functional position. Again, surgery should not be considered until at least 6 months after the sentinel event.

TBI

The most common causes of TBI in the population are motor vehicle collisions and gunshot wounds. Because of this situation, acquired spasticity caused by TBI is generally seen in the younger trauma population. Usually, they are younger individuals who survive the initial insult, and they often have foot ankle deformities that need to be addressed from a rehabilitation standpoint. Injury to the brain may be the result of a direct blow or an ischemic event. Ischemic damage may be focal as a result of a traumatic event or global from an anoxic event.

The patient who sustains a neurologic injury to the lateral cortex appears much the same as the patient with hemiplegia secondary to CVA. The issues of cognitive impairment, motor function, and sensibility require the same thorough evaluation as they do in patients with CVA. The key difference between younger patients with TBI and the older population with CVA is in the recovery period. The recovery period in the brain-injured patient is more variable, and improvement may still be noted 2 to 3 years after initial event. This longer recovery period stretches out the phase of mobilization and prevention of contractures and subsequent deformity and dysfunction.

Postpolio syndrome

Postpolio syndrome is the onset of new symptoms in survivors with documented acute poliomyelitis. Polio is caused by viral destruction of the anterior horn cells in the spinal cord and brain stem, the hallmark of which is preserved sensation with motor weakness. Postpolio syndrome results from long-term substitutions for muscle weakness that places increased demands on joints, ligaments, and muscles, and usually presents many years after the initial viral attack.[36,37] Postpolio syndrome is seen in approximately one-quarter of all former patients with polio. Several theories have been proposed for this late recurrence, but the most accepted explanation is overuse.[36] The most common symptoms include slowly progressive muscle weakness, fatigue, and muscle atrophy. Pain from joint degeneration and increasing skeletal deformities such as scoliosis can also occur. Survivors of polio are found to experience weakness, fatigue, and pain many years after their diagnosis, and the patients often complain that the muscles of their thigh tend to be tired, which in turn leads to aching and cramping. In the recovery phase, the return of strength is believed to result from adaptation at the neuromuscular junction, or, possibly, from muscle hypertrophy. Historically, recovery from this condition has been relatively successful, and survivors have resumed relatively functional lifestyles.

Evaluation The most common foot deformity of postpolio patients is a valgus hindfoot with midfoot collapse. With respect to evaluation, weakness of the calf muscles and limited ability of the quadriceps is difficult to appreciate because the signs of impairment are subtle. The signs of late weakness of the calf can be seen in the inability of the patient to perform 20 full range heel rises. When the patient is walking, persistent heel contact during the second half of the single stance phase is a basic indication of weakness.

The patient does not have the ability to support their body weight on the forefoot before the other foot strikes the ground, and increased dorsiflexion of the ankle becomes visible. However, in the setting of this muscular weakness, the patient does not have any sensory deficit. To address specific musculature, the most common area of weakness below the knee is the triceps surae. This deficit produces a calcaneal gait, which is defined by inability to push off but also instability as the weight progresses from hindfoot to midfoot. With a plantigrade foot and good ankle motion, a hinged ankle-foot orthosis with 5° to 10° of dorsiflexion and free plantar flexion allows the foot and ankle to toe off. Also, the use of this boot prevents overuse of the quadriceps during the early portion of the gait cycle.[36] Arthrodesis of the joints at the ankle, hindfoot, and midfoot should be considered when orthotic management has failed either to relieve symptoms in arthritic joints or to provide stability.[38]

Parkinson disease
Parkinson disease is a progressive, neurodegenerative disorder that is characterized by preferential degeneration of dopaminergic neurons in the substantia nigra pars compacta, and the presence of cytoplasmic inclusions known as Lewy bodies. Clinically, the patient has a resting tremor, bradykinesia, and rigidity. Parkinson disease is estimated at 0.3% of the entire population and 1% of the population older than 60 years.[39] It is an age-related disease, and the prevalence of the disease increases up to the ninth decade.

Workup The most distinctive clinical feature of physical examination is the resting tremor. Examination of motor tone reveals cogwheel rigidity in the affected limb. Examination of gait shows decreased arm swing on the affected side, small steps, and an inability to pivot and turn. Deep tendon reflexes and sensation are not affected. In addressing the foot and ankle, foot dystonia is the most common clinical finding in Parkinson disease,[40] and at least one-third of patients are affected with foot findings. If left untreated, the foot presents with plantar flexion of the ankle and supination at the subtalar joint, with plantar flexion of the lesser toes and extension of the hallux. Treatment of Parkinson disease with levodopa therapy may help with all of the patient's symptoms, except for that of the dystonic foot, and this medication may increase the severity of the spasms.[2,41–43] Because of the treatment, the foot dystonia is rarely a fixed contracture, and the primary orthopedic concern is prevention of a fixed deformity and enhancement of balance.

SUMMARY

Neuromuscular disorders of the foot and ankle are important to recognize, understand, and accurately diagnose. It is essential to determine the functional goals of the patient during the workup and particularly treatment planning stages. Accurate diagnosis, and informed discussion of treatment options, must be in the context of the patient's disease, cognition, comorbidities, functional attributes, and family environment. Regardless of cause, a thorough history and physical examination aid in an appropriate diagnostic workup and optimal orthopedic management of each patient.

REFERENCES

1. Mann RA. Examination of the foot and ankle. In: Mann RA, Coughlin MJ, editors. Surgery of the foot and ankle. St Louis (MO): Mosby; 1999. p. 36–51.
2. Mackenzie WG, Bowen JR. Muscle and nerve disorders in children. In: Chapman MW, editor. Chapman's orthopaedic surgery. 3rd edition. Philadelphia: Lippincott Williams & Wilkins; 2001. p. 4506–53.
3. Mankey MG. Peripheral nerve lesions of the foot and ankle. In: Chapman MW, editor. Chapman's orthopaedic surgery. 3rd edition. Philadelphia: Lippincott Williams & Wilkins; 2001. p. 3036–56.
4. Rab GT, Salamon PB. Congenital deformities of the foot. In: Chapman MW, editor. Chapman's orthopaedic surgery. 3rd edition. Philadelphia: Lippincott Williams & Wilkins; 2001. p. 4260–77.
5. Mayans D, Cartwright MS, Walker FO. Neuromuscular ultrasonography: quantifying muscle and nerve measurements. Phys Med Rehabil Clin N Am 2012; 23(1):133–48, xii.
6. Wnez W, Dreher T. Charcot-Marie-Tooth disease and the cavovarus foot. In: Pinzur MS, editor. Orthopaedic knowledge update 4, foot and ankle. Rosemont (IL): American Academy of Orthopaedic Surgeons. p. 291–307.
7. Espinós C, Calpena E, Martínez-Rubio D, et al. Autosomal recessive Charcot-Marie-Tooth neuropathy. Adv Exp Med Biol 2012;724:61–75.
8. Lupski JR, de Oca-Luna RM, Slaugenhaupt S, et al. DNA duplication associated with Charcot-Marie-Tooth disease type 1A. Cell 1991;66(2):219–32.
9. Beals T, Nickisch F. Charcot-Marie-Tooth Disease and the cavovarus foot. Foot Ankle Clin 2008;13:259–74.
10. Paulos L, Coleman SS, Samuelson KM. Pes cavovarus. Review of a surgical approach using selective soft-tissue procedures. J Bone Joint Surg Am 1980; 62(6):942–53.
11. Daher YU, Lonstein JE, Winter RB, et al. Spinal deformities in patients with Charcot-Marie-tooth disease. A review of 12 patients. Clin Orthop Relat Res 1986;(202): 219–22.
12. Sabir M, Lyttle D. Pathogenesis of Charcot-Marie-Tooth disease. Gait analysis and electrophysiologic, genetic, histopathologic, and enzyme studies in a kinship. Clin Orthop Relat Res 1984;(184):223–35.

13. Aiona MD, Leet AI. Neuromuscular disorders in children. In: Flynn J, editor. Ortho-paedic knowledge update 10. Rosemont (IL): American Academy of Orthopaedic Surgeons; 2011. p. 811–24.
14. Mann RA, Missirian J. Pathophysiology of Charcot-Marie-Tooth disease. Clin Orthop Relat Res 1988;(234):221–8.
15. Tynan MC, Klenerman L. The modified Robert Jones tendon transfer in cases of pes cavus and clawed hallux. Foot Ankle Int 1994;15(2):68–71.
16. Holmes JR, Hansen ST Jr. Foot and ankle manifestations of Charcot-Marie-Tooth disease. Foot Ankle 1993;14(8):476–86.
17. Skyre H. Genetic and clinical aspects of Charcot-Marie-Tooth's disease. Clin Genet 1974;6:98–118.
18. Dehne R. Congenital and acquired neurologic disorders. In: Mann RA, Coughlin MJ, editors. Surgery of the foot and ankle. St Louis (MO): Mosby; 1999. p. 525–60.
19. Coleman SS, Chesnut WJ. A simple test for hindfoot flexibility in the cavovarus foot. Clin Orthop Relat Res 1977;(123):60–2.
20. Gallardo E, Garcia A, Combarros O, et al. Charcot-Marie-Tooth disease type 1A duplication: spectrum of clinical and magnetic resonance imaging features in leg and foot muscles. Brain 2006;129(Pt 2):426–37.
21. Sharrard WJ, Grosfield I. The management of deformity and paralysis of the foot in myelomeningocele. J Bone Joint Surg Br 1968;50(3):456–65.
22. Beaty JH. Congenital foot deformities. In: Coughlin MJ, Mann RA, editors. Surgery of the foot and ankle. 8th edition. Philadelphia: Elsevier; 2006. p. 1729–60.
23. Gerlach DJ, Gurnett CA. Early results of the Ponseti method for treatment of the clubfoot associated with myelomeningocele. JBJS American 2009;91(6):1350–9.
24. van Mulken JM, Bulstra SK, Hoefnagels NH. Evaluation of the treatment of club-feet with the Diméglio score. J Pediatr Orthop 2001;21(5):642–7.
25. Shaheen S, Jaiballa H, Pirani S. Interobserver reliability in Pirani clubfoot severity scoring between a paediatric orthopaedic surgeon and a physiotherapy assis-tant. J Pediatr Orthop B 2012;21(4):366–8.
26. Eastwood DM. The clubfoot: congenital talipes equinovarus. In: Benson M, Fixen J, Macnicol M, et al, editors. Children's orthopaedics and fractures. 3rd edition. London: Springer; 2009. p. 541–58.
27. Robb JE, Brunner R. Orthopaedic management of cerebral palsy. In: Benson M, Fixen J, Macnicol M, et al, editors. Children's orthopaedics and fractures. 3rd edi-tion. London: Springer; 2009. p. 307–25.
28. Nelson KB, Ellenberg JH. Obstetric complications as risk factors for cerebral palsy or seizure disorders. JAMA 1984;251(14):1843–8.
29. Dehne R. Congenital and acquired neurologic deformities. In: Coughlin, Mann, editors. Surgery of the foot and ankle. 8th edition. 2006. p. 1761–807.
30. Minns RA. Neuromotor development and examination. In: Benson M, Fixen J, Macnicol M, et al, editors. Children's orthopaedics and fractures. 3rd edition. Lon-don: Springer; 2009. p. 231–48.
31. Drennan JC, Sharrad WJ. The pathologic anatomy of convex pes valgus. J Bone Joint Surg Br 1971;53(3):455–61.
32. Jordan C. Current status of functional lower extremity surgery in adult spastic pa-tients. Clin Orthop Relat Res 1988;(233):102–9.
33. Mooney V, Perry J, Nickel VL. Surgical and non-surgical orthopaedic care of stroke. J Bone Joint Surg Am 1967;49(5):989–1000.
34. Hickey JV, Todd AQ. Stroke. In: Hickey JV, editor. Clinical practice of neurological and neurosurgical nursing. Philadelphia: Lippincott Williams & Wilkins; 2009. p. 588–619.

35. Olney SJ, Richards C. Hemiparetic gait following stroke. Part I: characteristics. Gait Posture 1996;4(2):136–48.
36. Perry J, Fontaine JD, Mulroy S. Findings in post-poliomyelitis syndrome. Weakness of muscles of the calf as a source of late pain and fatigue of muscles of the thigh after poliomyelitis. J Bone Joint Surg Am 1995;77(8):1148–53.
37. Yarnell S. Poliomyelitis: the battle continues. JAMA 1990;261:3294–5.
38. Schaap EJ, Huy J, Tonino AJ. Long-term results of arthrodesis of the ankle. Int Orthop 1990;14(1):9–12.
39. De Lau LM, Breteler MM. Epidemiology of Parkinson's disease. Lancet Neurol 2006;5(6):525–35.
40. Lee RG, Tonolli I, Viallet F, et al. Preparatory postural adjustments in parkinsonian patients with postural instability. Can J Neurol Sci 1995;22:126–35.
41. Vidahet M, Bonnet AM, Marconi R, et al. Do parkinsonian symptoms and levodopa-induced dyskinesias start in the foot? Neurology 1994;44(9):1613–6.
42. Wukich D. Neurologic disorders of the foot and ankle. In: Lieberman JR, editor. AAOS comprehensive orthopaedic review. Rosemont (IL): American Academy of Orthopaedic Surgeons; 2009. p. 1225–38.
43. Bleck EE, Robb JE. Hereditary and developmental neuromuscular disorders. In: Benson M, Fixen J, Macnicol M, et al, editors. Children's orthopaedics and fractures. 3rd edition. London: Springer; 2009. p. 249–64.

Tendon Transfers—How Do They Work? Planning and Implementation

Thomas Dowd, MD[a], Eric M. Bluman, MD, PhD[b],*

KEYWORDS

- Tendon suspension • Interface • Balance • Fixation • Tension • Transplantation

KEY POINTS

- It is of utmost importance to match the patient's needs and goals with a well-planned procedure.
- Tendon transfers are optimally performed within a healthy soft tissue bed, across stable, mobile joints.
- The surgeon should seek to optimize motor unit characteristics (strength, excursion, expendability, direction of pull, phase, and integrity).
- A tendon transfer will result in optimized function with optimized muscle-tendon length restoration and insertion location.
- Perioperative treatment decisions have a direct impact on the tendon transfer success and proper selection will enhance the outcome.

INTRODUCTION

Tendon transfers are performed for a variety of conditions specific to the foot and ankle. They are suitable for addressing deformity, establishing, reestablishing, or augmenting motor function, or producing a tenodesis effect. These procedures are especially effective for correcting supple deformities caused by dynamic muscular imbalance.[1]

Five early stated principles were:

1. Restore the normal relationship between tendon and sheath.
2. Have the tendon course through tissue that is adapted to gliding of the tendon.
3. Imitate normal insertion of the tendon.
4. Establish normal tension.
5. Create an effective line of traction.[2]

[a] Foot and Ankle Service, Department of Orthopaedics and Rehabilitation, San Antonio Military Medical Center, 3551 Roger Brooke Dr., Fort Sam Houston, TX 78234, USA;
[b] Orthopedic Surgery, Harvard Medical School, Boston, MA 02115, USA
* Corresponding author.
E-mail address: ebluman@partners.org

Foot Ankle Clin N Am 19 (2014) 17–27
http://dx.doi.org/10.1016/j.fcl.2013.10.003
1083-7515/14/$ – see front matter Published by Elsevier Inc.

foot.theclinics.com

Based on these tenets, a variety of orthopedic specialties have used a multitude of tendon transfer procedures. Despite many generations of widespread clinical use, there remains a lack of definitive evidence as guidance toward their optimal performance.

This article provides an update on the literature from all orthopedic subspecialties in an effort to present applicable data that may be used to inform optimal performance of tendon transfers about the foot and ankle.

NOMENCLATURE

A variety of terms have been used to describe those procedures by which motor units are surgically modified to improve function. It is worth reviewing the terms and their definitions to minimize confusion (**Table 1**).

PLANNING AND PERFORMING TENDON TRANSFERS

The performance of tendon transfers should be individually tailored to the specific needs of each patient. Nevertheless, established guidelines should be followed in the planning and performance of these procedures. Certain prerequisites must be met before undertaking the actual tendon transfer. After meeting the appropriate criteria, there are 5 basic principles that should guide the selection of the optimal motor for balance between the transfer muscle and its antagonist muscles. These principles include restoration of a normal tendon-sheath relationship, coursing the tendon through tissue that will permit gliding, re-creating the normal tendon insertion, establishing normal tension, and creating an effective line of traction.[2] After prerequisites are met and basic principles are followed, additional factors should be considered and are also discussed.

Prerequisites for Successful Tendon Transfer

Analysis of the patient's needs and goals

As with any surgical treatment, the goals of the intervention should match patient needs. The patient should be aware of what improvements in function can reasonably be expected and how the procedure is intended to help meet stated goals. In addition, it is important to review any limitations that might result from the transfer of a currently functioning tendon. The specific advantages and disadvantages should be emphasized and patient understanding confirmed before proceeding with any intervention.

Table 1
Delineation of Different Tendon Procedures

Type	Description	Example
Tendon transfer	Relocation of tendon insertion to a new site[6]	Flexor digitorum longus tendon to posterior tibial tendon insertion
Tendon translocation	Rerouting of tendon without disruption of origin or insertion	Young procedure to reroute the anterior tibial tendon for adult acquired flatfoot disorder[7,8]
Muscle tendon transplantation	Entire motor unit is detached and implanted in new location	Rectus femoris, gracilis, and latissimus dorsi transfers[9,10]
Tendon suspension (tenosuspension)	Rerouting of a tendon to create support for a structure[11]	Jones and Hibbs tenosuspensions[12]

Adequate soft tissue bed for coverage

Owing to the limited soft tissue envelope often encountered about the foot and ankle, adequate soft tissue coverage is essential. Transfers performed without adequate coverage will become desiccated, infected, or both. Weaves used for fixation increase the effective tendon volume and may lead to problems with incisional closure or healing. Although it is important to consider what is being covered, it is of equal importance to consider what is available for coverage. If the soft tissue available for coverage is highly scarred or contracted, tendon transfer may be contraindicated.

Mobile intercalary joints

The purposes of tendon transfers—correction of deformity, improvement of motor function, and creation of a tenodesis effect—cannot be accomplished without mobile joints. If the intended tendon transfer cannot act on a mobile joint, it should not be performed.

Bony and joint stability

Although tendon transfers require mobile joints to bring about their intended function, stability is also required at the intervening bones and joints. Tendon transfers spanning unstable nonunions will be at best suboptimal, may accentuate deformity, or have less than their desired function. In similar fashion, some degree of joint stability is requisite. A transfer acting on an articulation without any stability will fail. Tendon transfer should attempt augment existing joint stability rather than be relied on to exclusively provide stability.

Donor motor unit qualities

Several different criteria should be met for an optimally functioning transfer. Consideration needs to be given that there will be some loss of strength encountered with each tendon transfer. This loss of strength will be acceptable as long as there is adequate residual strength to perform the required action. Lack of excursion may result in limited function because of gradually decreased motion and eventual joint contractures. The donor site from which the tendon is transferred will lose strength, function, or both. Essential functions must not be sacrificed. Any gain of function must outweigh any loss resulting from transfer. Transfer of an antagonist muscle not only weakens of the antagonistic function but also augments the desired function.

The basic principles for successful tendon transfer are summarized in **Table 2**.

Other Technical Considerations

Tensioning

There is a relationship between the tension at which a tendon transfer is set and the strength of the muscle transfer. There exists controversy regarding the proper tension at which to set a tendon transfer.[3] Tensioning errors have been cited as a cause of poor outcomes in certain procedures.[4]

A muscle fiber responds differently under passive and active conditions. On passive lengthening, a muscle acts much like an elastic band: The more the fiber is stretched, the more tension is realized until the point of failure (rupture). However, this linear relationship is not preserved when looking at the active tension able to be generated by a muscle in relationship to changes to the resting length of muscle (as demonstrated by the Blix curve).[5]

At the histologic level, the relationship between length and tension generated is defined by the degree of actin-myosin overlap within the sarcomere. At resting length nearly all of the myosin heads are in contact with actin. When the muscle fiber is stimulated to fire, maximal tension is generated because of this optimal overlap. As the

Table 2
Principles of Tendon Transfers

Principle	Explanation	Determination
Strength	Enough force generated to perform desired activity	Cross-sectional area
Amplitude	Magnitude of excursion adequate for desired function	Clinical and intraoperative testing
Direction	Line of pull should be as straight as possible	Evaluation of anatomic path after transfer
Attachment	Use of offset from joint center of rotation to set appropriate force generated	Chose insertion site to provide adequate force without causing bowstringing
Synergy		
Phase	Transferred tendon's normal contractile period (eg, swing, push off) should be the same as that trying to be augmented	Goal to have muscle contract during expected motion
Integrity	Transfer should have single function	Make sure all components of transfer act to create a balanced and concerted motion; multiple transfers should have matched excursion

muscle lengthens beyond its resting length, this overlap starts to diminish and the resulting tension capability decreases. Similarly, if the starting length is less than the resting length, the myosin is not able to optimally progress along the actin filament and less tension is realized.

Formation of a Stable Bone-Tendon Interface

It is important to create a stable attachment of the tendon to bone for long-term proper functioning of a tendon transfer. Studies have been performed on the optimization of this interface for more than 70 years and continue today.

Early works sought to define the process of the attachment of tendon transfers to bone, focusing on the histologic maturation at the interface between the 2 structures.[6–8] In recent years, Rodeo and colleagues[9] have enhanced the understanding of the maturation of tendon transfers to bone. Through their animal studies, 3 phases have been identified in this process. The first phase occurs in the first 2 weeks following the procedure and involves the formation of fibrovascular tissue at the tendon-bone interface. The second phase proceeds between 2 and 12 weeks, with development of a thin seam of new bone along the bone tunnel with a diminishment in vascularity compared with the 2-week specimens. There is occasional continuity of collagen fibers from bone to the tendon. Twelve weeks after transfer, there is increased maturation of the interface tissue with fibers starting to align themselves along the direction of pull of the tendon. At 26 weeks following tendon transfer into bone, there is increased alignment of the collagen fibers along the direction of pull of the tendon throughout the length of the tendon. There is also remodeling of the trabecular bone surrounding the tendon. The last phase is maturation of tendon-bone interface.

It seems that approximately 3 months is required after tendon transfer for a stable bone-tendon interface to be formed. Rodeo and colleagues[9] performed biomechanical testing to evaluate temporal strength changes. During the first 8 weeks after tendon implantation, all specimens failed by pullout of the tendon at the bone-tendon interface. By 12 weeks, the interface had strengthened so that failure occurred along the course of the tendon proper. There was no further functional maturation of this interface past 12 weeks.

Tendon Anchoring

Several different methods have been successfully used to secure tendon to bone. Early methods of fixation included passing the tendon through a bone tunnel and then suturing it back on itself. This method requires an adequate length of tendon and a location at which it is possible to turn the tendon back on itself. Another method that can be used when it is difficult to suture the tendon on itself is to pass the tendon through a bone tunnel and secure it to a button on the skin.[10] Several commercial devices have also been developed to strengthen fixation or provide fixation alternatives when tendon length is limited. These devices include staples,[11] spiked washers,[12] bone anchors,[13] soft tissue interference screws,[14] and adjustable suture suspension within bone.[15] Although these devices may increase the initial fixation strength, they are not without limitations. Both spiked washer and staple use have been associated with soft tissue necrosis and the eventual fixation may be more dependent on the ensuing inflammatory response than the friction between the tendon and the implant.[12,16] However, the clinical impact of this concern is uncertain.

Soft tissue interference screws were originally constructed from titanium. These screws were found to have the unacceptable complication of occasionally lacerating the tendon graft.[17] Bioabsorbable screws demonstrated adequate fixation with minimal damage to the graft. These screws have been fashioned from poly-L-lactic acid and bone dowels and have become the choice of surgeons using soft tissue interference screws in recent years. Less traumatic, nonabsorbable screws have also been fashioned from polyetheretherketone and are now commercially available.[18]

Scranton and colleagues[19] looked at suture anchor fixation in cadaveric bone. Differences in insertion technique yielded varying results. Anchors composed of plastic failed at the eyelet. They concluded that if suture anchors are used at least 2 should be placed for each anchor point.[19] The angle of suture anchor insertion also influences pullout strength. Burkhart and colleagues[20] showed that the "deadman's angle" allows the threads of the anchor and the structure of the surrounding bone to combine to maximize pullout strength of these devices. This angle of the insertion is such that the inserted point of the bone anchor is canted approximately 45° toward the direction of pull of the tendon. Although the model for testing is not without controversy, this subject has been revisited with evidence to suggest that suture anchor insertion at 90° relative to the direction of pull may result in increased strength of fixation.[21]

Sullivan and colleagues[22] compared the strength of suture anchor fixation to sewing the tendon to itself when transferring the flexor digitorum longus to the medial navicular. They demonstrated that the mean load to failure was nearly identical for each group.[22] The downside to the latter technique is the increased length of tendon required, although the cost incurred with use of a suture anchor is greatly increased. A similar experimental design was used by Sabonghy and colleagues,[14] but using soft tissue interference screws rather than suture anchors. This group found that sewing the tendon to itself was stronger than using a soft tissue interference screw, but both provided enough strength at the bone-tendon interface to counteract physiologic forces encountered by tendons.

A recent study demonstrated increased strength of fixation using a soft tissue interference screw as compared with a bone anchor in an in vitro model of the split anterior tendon transfer.[23] Suture suspension devices and bone anchors involve additional sites of interface (bone/device, device/suture, suture/tendon), which may predispose the transferred tendon to weakness or elongation. Although the soft tissue interference screw fixation was significantly stronger, it is unknown whether this translates into a clinical difference. A study with a similar design looking at fixation strength for an autograft lateral ankle ligament reconstruction showed that the soft tissue interference screw was significantly stronger in fixing the tendon to bone than bone anchors. The values obtained for the soft tissue interference screws seem to be greater than the values for load to failure of the native anterior talofibular ligament.[24]

The appropriate size tunnel to use with interference screw fixation was examined by Louden and colleagues.[25] In this study, pilot hole diameter was varied for 2 different sizes of interference screws to determine which provided better fixation strength. The authors noted that there was a significant difference in pullout strength between 7-mm and 5-mm screws, but the pilot hole size did not influence the pullout strength for a given screw size. Greater than adequate fixation was obtained with both screw sizes irrespective of pilot hole size even in poor quality bone.

Location

Classic teaching has been that tendon transfers will heal better to a raw bleeding cancellous surface than to intact cortical bone. One example is the belief that for proper healing rotator cuff repairs must be secured into a cancellous trough at the greater tuberosity of the humerus.[26,27] The exact rationale for this teaching is not known, but likely arose from the belief that the interface that forms between a tendon and cancellous bone is biomechanically superior to that formed between a tendon and cortical bone. St Pierre and colleagues[28] tested this assumption in an in vivo animal model of rotator cuff repair. They compared the biomechanical properties of infraspinatus repairs affixed with a cortical trough to those repaired directly to cancellous bone. Interestingly, there was no difference in the strength of repairs in the load to failure, energy to failure, or stiffness between the 2 groups at 6 and 12 weeks after the repair.[28]

Biologics and Physiologic Factors

The study of biologics and biologic response modifiers in relation to tendon transfers is in its infancy. Although several different biologics have been investigated, the number of studies performed is low. Some of the substances studied are not available commercially but have been included for completeness.

Researchers have assessed the impact of wrapping periosteum around tendon ends inserted into bone. A variety of rabbit model studies has been performed and all have demonstrated improved strength of fixation with use of periosteal tendon wraps.[29–31]

A recent review of the potential mechanisms of periosteal enhancement of tendon-bone healing suggests that periosteal tendon wraps offer an excellent source of progenitor cells, local growth factor source, and scaffold for the cells and factors. Furthermore, the addition of the periosteum may improve the initial mechanical fixation.[32]

Bone morphogenetic proteins are growth factors that induce bone formation in tissues with the capacity to do so.[33] An in vivo animal study has demonstrated that bone morphogenetic protein-2 is able to augment tendon healing to bone.[34] This study was performed in a 2-stage model in which an ossicle was generated within the tendon to be transferred and this tendon-ossicle complex was then fixed to the recipient site. With this model, higher ultimate load to failure values were observed after healing. However, it is unclear whether such a 2-stage approach could be practically adopted in clinical practice. A recent animal study demonstrated that the local application of bone morphogenetic protein-2 to a tendon-bone interference site resulted in increased osteoid formation at 3 weeks, but no improvement in mechanical properties.[35]

Receptor activator of nuclear factor-KB; ligand stimulates osteoclast formation in cells of the monocyte lineage. It also has direct catabolic effects on bone and has been shown to reduce bone density, volume, and strength.[36] Because of these findings, it was thought that the receptor activator of nuclear factor-KB; ligand would diminish the tendon-bone interface. However, its addition did not decrease the histologic or biomechanical properties of the bone-tendon interface compared with control specimens. Osteoprotegerin is a soluble receptor antagonist to the receptor activator of nuclear factor-KB;. Because it antagonizes osteoclast formation, it augments the maturation of the bone-tendon interface.[37]

Platelet concentrates also modulate tendon-to-bone healing. Addition of platelet concentrate alone to hamstring anterior cruciate ligament reconstruction led to uniform magnetic resonance imaging evidence of graft incorporation within a bone tunnel at 6 months that was significantly improved over a control group. However, no functionally statistical differences in the groups were found.[38] A recent review of the effect of platelet concentrates demonstrated a variable, 20% to 30% average benefit to graft maturation, whereas there is limited evidence to suggest improved tendon-bone healing. Indeed, there has yet to be demonstrated a difference in clinical outcome with the use of platelet concentrates.[39]

One group has tested a magnesium-based bone adhesive for repairing flexor tendons to bone in an animal model. They found that the initial biomechanical properties of these repairs are improved with the adhesive, but in vivo use led to a decrease in the strength of the repair.[40] Presently, the use of these adhesives cannot be recommended.

Nonsteroidal Anti-Inflammatory Drugs

The effect of nonsteroidal anti-inflammatory drug (NSAID) use on tendon-bone healing has been investigated.[41–43] Most recently, Dimmen and colleagues[42] showed that the development of a strong interface relative to untreated control animals was delayed in those exposed to NSAIDs. In the study animals, 3 groups were tested for strength to pullout. There were 2 study groups that received either parecoxib or indomethacin after Achilles tendon transplant into the tibia. The control group did not receive any NSAID. Both experimental groups showed significantly diminished interface strength as compared with the control group.[42] A recent study evaluated the effect of ibuprofen on the expression of matrix metalloproteinases and collagen. Metalloproteinases 1, 8, 9, and 13 were up-regulated by this NSAID, whereas type 1 and 3 collagen expression was not affected, suggesting that ibuprofen may have an inhibitory effect on tendon healing.[44]

Nicotine

Although the detrimental effects of nicotine on fracture healing and joint fusion have been well described, little is known about its effect on the healing of soft tissues such as tendon and ligament. In an in vivo model of healing of rotator cuff to bone, Galatz and colleagues[45] demonstrated that the rotator cuff attachment of animals exposed to nicotine had decreased maximum stress and maximum force relative to those in the control group. They also demonstrated that cellular proliferation and type I collagen expression were lower in the nicotine-treated animals relative to controls. Inflammation persisted longer in the nicotine-treated animals.

The authors surmised that these findings may at least partly explain the inferior biomechanical properties demonstrated by the nicotine-treated groups.[45] Recent work has evaluated the dose effect of nicotine on the supraspinatus in a rat model. Contrary to expectations, nicotine exposure was noted to result in a trend toward increased maximum stress and maximum load before failure. However, the modulus of elasticity was increased, which has been associated with increased risk of rupture.[46]

Immobilization/Mobilization

Tendons and their surrounding tissues respond to mechanical changes in their environment. In general, increased loads across these structures lead to increases in their tensile modulus, whereas decreases in applied stress cause a diminution in their mechanical properties.

Studies on early loading of tendon grafts have been contradictory. One previous study demonstrated that the strength of graft integration of rabbit anterior cruciate ligament repairs was impaired in animals allowed unlimited cage activity.[47] Another showed that early exercise compromised healing of an animal rotator cuff repair model. However, Thomopoulos and colleagues[48] have subsequently demonstrated that muscle loading after canine flexor tendon repair improved the biomechanical properties compared with animals whose repairs went unloaded. Bedi and colleagues[49] showed that early delayed application of cyclic axial loads increased load to failure, new bone formation, tissue mineral content, and density at the tendon-bone interface. The load to failure was highest in animals that had daily applied loads started 4 days postoperatively.[49]

More recently, Brophy and colleagues identified no strength difference at the bone-tendon interface in ACL-reconstructed rats between immobilized and short-duration, low-magnitude cyclic loading groups. However, the cyclic loading group did demonstrate increased inflammation and decreased bone formation.[50] Interestingly, these investigators also recently demonstrated paradoxic findings with respect to immobilization of native and repaired tendons at 2 and 4 weeks. At 2 weeks, the native, immobilized tendon was stronger compared with its repaired counterpart. However, 4 weeks of immobilization resulted in significant weakening of the native tendon, resulting in significant weakness as compared with the repaired tendons. It is difficult to compare these heterogeneous studies but they provide a useful foundation for further research and data to help guide the transition from immobilization to return of motion.

SUMMARY

Tendon transfers are powerful procedures that, when properly applied, have demonstrated the ability to restore substantial function. There are important procedural considerations and inherent limitations to acknowledge before the use of these techniques. It is paramount to match the patient's needs and goals with the appropriate procedure. Tendon transfers are optimally performed within a healthy soft tissue bed, across stable, mobile joints, and using motor unit characteristics (strength, excursion, expendability, direction of pull, phase, and integrity). Special attention must be paid to proper tension and insertion location. the perioperative care should include appropriate immobilization, subsequent rehabilitation, analgesics, and avoidance of nicotine. As this field evolves, especially with respect to adjunctive treatments, an informed surgeon will optimize the outcome when tendon transfers are used in the treatment of musculoskeletal conditions.

REFERENCES

1. Peabody C. Tendon transposition. J Bone Joint Surg Am 1938;20:193.
2. Bluman EM, Dowd T. The basics and science of tendon transfers. Foot Ankle Clin 2011;16(3):385–99.
3. Mayer L. The physiologic method of tendon transplantation.I. Historical, anatomy and physiology of tendons. Surg Gynecol Obstet 1916;22:182–97.
4. Piazza SJ, Adamson RL, Moran MF, et al. Effects of tensioning errors in split transfers of tibialis anterior and posterior tendons. J Bone Joint Surg Am 2003;85(5):858–65.
5. Blix M. Die Lange und die Spannung des Muskels. Skand Arch Physiol 1895;5: 173–206.
6. Kernwein G. Tendon implantations to bone: a study of the factors affecting tendon-bone union as determined by the tensile strength. Ann Surg 1941;113:1103.
7. Whiston TB, Walmsley R. Some observations on the reactions of bone and tendon after tunnelling of bone and insertion of tendon. J Bone Joint Surg Br 1960;42:377.
8. Forward AD, Cowan RJ. Experimental suture of tendon to bone. Surg Forum 1960;11:458.
9. Rodeo SA, Arnoczky SP, Torzilli PA, et al. Tendon-healing in a bone tunnel. A biomechanical and histological study in the dog. J Bone Joint Surg Am 1993; 75:1795.
10. Key JA. Fixation of tendons, ligaments and bone by Bunnell's pull-out wire suture. Ann Surg 1946;123:656.
11. Goh JC, Lee PY, Lee EH, et al. Biomechanical study on tibialis posterior tendon transfers. Clin Orthop Relat Res 1995;319:297.
12. Straight CB, France EP, Paulos LE, et al. Soft tissue fixation to bone. A biomechanical analysis of spiked washers. Am J Sports Med 1994;22:339.
13. Myerson MS, Cohen I, Uribe J. An easy way of tensioning and securing a tendon to bone. Foot Ankle Int 2002;23:753.
14. Sabonghy EP, Wood RM, Ambrose CG, et al. Tendon transfer fixation: comparing a tendon to tendon technique vs. bioabsorbable interference-fit screw fixation. Foot Ankle Int 2003;24:260.
15. Bluman EM. Technique tip: suture suspension of tendons. Foot Ankle Int 2007; 28:854.
16. Bargar WL, Sharkey NA, Paul HA, et al. Efficacy of bone staples for fixation. J Orthop Trauma 1987;1(4):326–30.
17. McGuire DA, Barber FA, Elrod BF, et al. Bioabsorbable interference screws for graft fixation in anterior cruciate ligament reconstruction. Arthroscopy 1999;15:463.
18. Nho SJ, Provencher MT, Seroyer ST, et al. Bioabsorbable anchors in glenohumeral shoulder surgery. Arthroscopy 2009;25:788.
19. Scranton PE Jr, Lawhon SM, McDermott JE. Bone suture anchor fixation in the lower extremity: a review of insertion principles and a comparative biomechanical evaluation. Foot Ankle Int 2005;26:516.
20. Burkhart SS, Lo IKY, Brady PC. Burkhart's view of the shoulder: a cowboy's guide to advanced shoulder arthroscopy. Philadelphia: Lippincott Williams & Wilkins; 2006.
21. Strauss E, Frank D, Kubiak E, et al. The effect of the angle of suture anchor insertion on fixation failure at the tendon-suture interface after rotator cuff repair: deadman's angle revisited. Arthroscopy 2009;25:597.

22. Sullivan RJ, Gladwell HA, Aronow MS, et al. An in vitro study comparing the use of suture anchors and drill hole fixation for flexor digitorum longus transfer to the navicular. Foot Ankle Int 2006;27:363.
23. Nunez-Pereira S, Pacha-Vicente D, Llusa-Perez M, et al. Tendon transfer fixation in the foot and ankle: a biomechanical study. Foot Ankle Int 2009;30:1207.
24. Jeys L, Korrosis S, Stewart T, et al. Bone anchors or interference screws? A biomechanical evaluation for autograft ankle stabilization. Am J Sports Med 2004;32:1651.
25. Louden KW, Ambrose CG, Beaty SG, et al. Tendon transfer fixation in the foot and ankle: a biomechanical study evaluating two sizes of pilot holes for bio-absorbable screws. Foot Ankle Int 2003;24:67.
26. Miller RH, Azar FM, Throckmorton TW. Shoulder and elbow injuries. In: Crenshaw AH, Daugherty K, Campbell WC, editors. Campbell's operative orthopaedics. 8th edition. St Louis (MO): Mosby Year Book; 1992. p. 2213–45.
27. Poppen N. Soft-tissue lesions of the shoulder. In: Chapman M, Madison M, editors. Operative orthopaedics. Philadelphia: Lippincott; 1988. p. 745.
28. St Pierre P, Olson EJ, Elliott JJ, et al. Tendon-healing to cortical bone compared with healing to a cancellous trough. A biomechanical and histological evaluation in goats. J Bone Joint Surg Am 1995;77:1858.
29. Ohtera K, Yamada Y, Aoki M, et al. Effects of periosteum wrapped around tendon in a bone tunnel: a biomechanical and histological study in rabbits. Crit Rev Biomed Eng 2000;28(1–2):115–8.
30. Youn I, Jones DG, Andrews PJ, et al. Periosteal augmentation of a tendon graft improves tendon healing in the bone tunnel. Clin Orthop Relat Res 2004;419:223–31.
31. Karaoglu S, Celik C, Korkusuz P. The effects of bone marrow or periosteum on tendon-to-bone tunnel healing in a rabbit model. Knee Surg Sports Traumatol Arthrosc 2009;17:170–8.
32. Li H, Jiang J, Wu Y, et al. Potential mechanisms of a periosteum patch as an effective and favourable approach to enhance tendon-bone healing in the human body. International Orthopaedics 2012;36(3):665.
33. Gautschi OP, Frey SP, Zellweger R. Bone morphogenetic proteins in clinical applica- tions. Aust N Z J Surg 2007;77:626.
34. Hashimoto Y, Yoshida G, Toyoda H, et al. Generation of tendon-to-bone interface "enthesis" with use of recombinant BMP-2 in a rabbit model. J Orthop Res 2007;25:1415.
35. Thomopoulos S, Kim HM, Silva MJ, et al. Effect of bone morphogenetic protein 2 on tendon-to-bone healing in a canine flexor tendon model. J Orthop Res 2012;30:1702–9.
36. Kostenuik PJ. Osteoprotegerin and RANKL regulate bone resorption, density, geometry and strength. Curr Opin Pharmacol 2005;5:618.
37. Rodeo SA, Kawamura S, Ma CB, et al. The effect of osteoclastic activity on tendon- to-bone healing: an experimental study in rabbits. J Bone Joint Surg Am 2007;89:2250.
38. Orrego M, Larrain C, Rosales J, et al. Effects of platelet concentrate and a bone plug on the healing of hamstring tendons in a bone tunnel. Arthroscopy 2008;24:1373.
39. Vavken P, Sadoghi P, Murray MM. The effect of platelet concentrates on graft maturation and graft-bone interface healing in anterior cruciate ligament reconstruction in human patients: a systematic review of controlled trials. Arthroscopy 2011;27(11):1573.

40. Thomopoulos S, Zampiakis E, Das R, et al. Use of a magnesium-based bone adhesive for flexor tendon-to-bone healing. J Hand Surg Am 2009;34:1066.

41. Cohen DB, Kawamura S, Ehteshami JR, et al. Indomethacin and celecoxib impair rotator cuff tendon-to-bone healing. Am J Sports Med 2006;34:362.

42. Dimmen S, Nordsletten L, Engebretsen L, et al. The effect of parecoxib and indo-metacin on tendon-to-bone healing in a bone tunnel: an experimental study in rats. J Bone Joint Surg Br 2009;91:259.

43. Ferry ST, Dahners LE, Afshari HM, et al. The effects of common anti-inflammatory drugs on the healing rat patellar tendon. Am J Sports Med 2007;35:1326.

44. Tsai WC, Hsu CC, Pang JH, et al. Ibuprofen upregulates expression of matrix metalloproteinase-1, -8, -9 and expressions of types I and III collagen in tendon cells. J Orthop Res 2010;28:487–91.

45. Galatz LM, Silva MJ, Rothermich SY, et al. Nicotine delays tendon-to-bone healing in a rat shoulder model. J Bone Joint Surg Am 2006;88:2027.

46. Ichinose R, Sano H, Itoi E, et al. Alteration of the material properties of the normal supraspinatus tendon by nicotine treatment in a rat model. Acta Orthopaedica 2010;81:634–8.

47. Sakai H, Fukui N, Kawakami A, et al. Biological fixation of the graft within bone after anterior cruciate ligament reconstruction in rabbits: effects of the duration of postoperative immobilization. J Orthop Sci 2000;5:43.

48. Thomopoulos S, Zampiakis E, Das R, et al. The effect of muscle loading on flexor tendon-to-bone healing in a canine model. J Orthop Res 2008;26:1611.

49. Bedi A, Kovacevic D, Fox AJ, et al. Effect of early and delayed mechanical loading on tendon-to-bone healing after anterior cruciate ligament reconstruction. J Bone Joint Surg Am 2010;92:2387–401.

50. Brophy RH, Kovacevic D, Rodeo SA, et al. Effect of short-duration low-magnitude cyclic loading versus immobilization on tendon-bone healing after ACL reconstruction in a rat model. J Bone Joint Surg Am 2011;93:381–93.

Tendon Transfers in the Treatment of the Adult Flatfoot

Jonathon D. Backus, MD[a], Jeremy J. McCormick, MD[b],*

KEYWORDS

- Adult acquired flatfoot deformity • Posterior tibial tendon dysfunction
- Tendon transfer • Tibialis posterior • Flexor digitorum longus • Flexor hallucis longus
- Peroneus brevis • Peroneus longus

KEY POINTS

- Adult acquired flatfoot deformity (AAFD) describes a condition of progressive hindfoot valgus, forefoot abduction, and forefoot varus. It is most commonly caused by posterior tibial tendon dysfunction.
- Patients who have AAFD often complain of posteromedial hindfoot pain, a progressive change in the shape of the foot, difficulty with weight bearing, and gait abnormalities.
- Conservative management consists of nonsteroidal antiinflammatory medications, selective corticosteroid injections, and physical therapy. Patients also benefit from temporary immobilization in a cast or boot, custom foot orthosis, or a custom ankle-foot orthosis or Arizona brace.
- In stage I and II posterior tibial tendon (PTT) dysfunction in which conservative management has failed, many clinicians think that the deformity can be corrected with PTT debridement, tendon transfer, and a medial displacement calcaneal osteotomy. Spring ligament repair may also be indicated in certain cases.
- In more significant stage II deformities, concomitant procedures such as an additional lateral column-lengthening osteotomy and selective fusions may be required.
- In the case of a stage II flexible flatfoot deformity, our preference is to excise the diseased PTT tendon and use a flexor digitorum longus (FDL) transfer through a tunnel in the navicular tuberosity. The FDL tendon is typically long enough to pass through the tunnel from plantar to dorsal and be secured back to itself with nonabsorbable suture.

Continued

Financial Disclosures: There are no financial relationships or support to disclose for J.D. Backus. Research funding was received from Wright Medical Technologies, Inc and Midwest Stone Institute, paid laboratory instructing for Synthes, Inc and Integra Life Sciences, Inc; there are no conflicts with relation to this article for J.J. McCormick.
[a] Department of Orthopaedic Surgery, Washington University School of Medicine in St Louis, Campus Box 8233, 660 South Euclid Avenue, St Louis, MO 63110, USA; [b] Department of Orthopaedic Surgery, Washington University School of Medicine in St Louis, 14532 South Outer Forty Drive, Suite 210, Chesterfield, MO 63017, USA
* Corresponding author.
E-mail address: mccormickj@wudosis.wustl.edu

Foot Ankle Clin N Am 19 (2014) 29–48
http://dx.doi.org/10.1016/j.fcl.2013.11.002
1083-7515/14/$ – see front matter © 2014 Elsevier Inc. All rights reserved.

Continued

- Patients with stage III and stage IV deformities typically require a hindfoot arthrodesis. A plantarflexion osteotomy or fusion of the first ray may also be required in patients with persistent forefoot varus. Furthermore, there may be a role for tendon transfer in patients who undergo hindfoot arthrodesis.
- The decision to proceed with surgical correction of AAFD should be made after conservative treatment options have failed. Careful preoperative planning is necessary to choose the appropriate reconstructive procedures given a patient's clinical examination, deformity, and radiographic findings.

PATHOPHYSIOLOGY OF ADULT ACQUIRED FLATFOOT DEFORMITY

Adult acquired flatfoot deformity (AAFD) describes a condition of progressive hindfoot valgus, forefoot abduction, and forefoot varus. Although there are several causes of AAFD, posterior tibial tendon (PTT) dysfunction is the most common cause.[1] The posterior tibialis (PT) muscle is a powerful supinator of the subtalar joint, adductor of the midfoot, and serves to assist plantar flexion of the ankle. It has 9 attachments to the medial midfoot that help this muscle statically support the arch of the foot along with the spring ligament and the plantar calcaneonavicular ligament.[2,3] Therefore, the PT muscle has important functions throughout the stance phase of gait and in the overall structure and function of the foot and ankle.

During the early part of stance phase, the PT muscle contracts eccentrically allowing the hindfoot to pronate in a controlled fashion and subsequently unlock the talonavicular and calcaneocuboid joints. This function allows the foot to become supple and adapt to the undulations of the underlying surface that it contacts. In toe-off, the muscle contracts concentrically, supinating the hindfoot and locking the talonavicular and calcaneocuboid joints, which provides a rigid fulcrum for the gastrocsoleus muscle to propel the body forward and begin the swing phase of gait.

In the early stages of PTT disorder, the dysfunctional tendon leaves the spring and calcaneonavicular ligaments unsupported in counteracting the antagonistic hindfoot pronation and forefoot abduction forces of the peroneus brevis (PB). The arch is usually maintained at first; however, with continued PTT dysfunction and the stress of ambulation, the spring ligament eventually fails and the arch gradually collapses.[4] Persistent hindfoot valgus and forefoot abduction eventually result in forefoot varus, which may manifest as dorsiflexion of the first ray or global forefoot varus at the transverse tarsal joint (**Fig. 1**).[5] At first, these deformities are flexible and passively correctable; however, consequent synovitis and scarring lead to the foot becoming fixed in its malpositioned posture.

SYMPTOMS

Patients with AAFD typically complain of posteromedial hindfoot pain below the medial malleolus, a progressive change in the shape of the foot, and difficulty with weight bearing; however, patients rarely report a specific instance in which the foot collapses. Some patients also experience lateral pain near the sinus tarsi if the deformity is such that the lateral malleolus impinges with the calcaneus.[6] Patients often note gait disturbances such as difficulty with push-off, long strides, and an inability to run.[7]

STAGING

Johnson and Strom[8] described the first classification system for PTT dysfunction and AAFD in 1998. This classification is helpful in that it is often used to determine

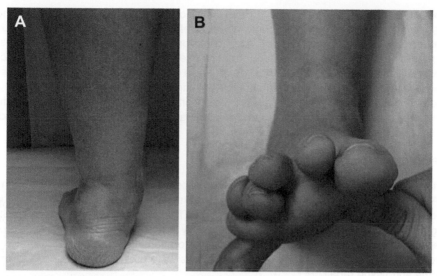

Fig. 1. (*A*) Preoperative assessment of hindfoot valgus. (*B*) Preoperative assessment of forefoot varus. (*Courtesy of* Jeffrey E. Johnson, MD, Chesterfield, MO.)

treatment. Stage I represents PT tendinitis and degeneration, with normal tendon length and an intact medial longitudinal arch. In stage II, the PTT elongates and a flexible flatfoot deformity develops. Stage III represents a flatfoot with fixed deformity. Myerson[9] added a 4th stage to Johnson and Strom's[8] classification that described deltoid ligament attenuation and a fixed valgus ankle deformity as a result of prolonged planovalgus foot deformity (**Table 1**).

CONSERVATIVE MANAGEMENT

Nonoperative treatment can be performed initially for a deformity of any stage; however, it is most effective for stage I and mild stage II deformities.[10] Initial treatment consists of nonsteroidal antiinflammatory medications, physical therapy, and a custom-molded orthosis. Clinicians can also prescribe a semirigid foot orthosis that is posted at the medial heel and lateral forefoot, which helps support the arch and

Table 1	
Classification system for PTT dysfunction	
Stage	**Clinical Finding**
I[8]	Pain along PTT Intact medial longitudinal arch Able to perform single-limb heel rise
II[8]	Loss of medial longitudinal arch (flatfoot) Unable to perform single-limb heel rise Hindfoot can be passively reduced to neutral posture
III[8]	Loss of medial longitudinal arch (flatfoot) Unable to perform single-limb heel rise Hindfoot cannot be passively reduced to neutral posture
IV[9]	Stage II or III findings with valgus posture at the ankle caused by deltoid insufficiency

correct hindfoot valgus and pronation with the medial heel post and arch support, and also corrects forefoot varus through lateral forefoot support. If the forefoot varus deformity is rigid, an accommodative semirigid orthosis with a medial forefoot post is recommended to support the forefoot in its fixed position. If an orthosis is unsuccessful or the patient has a more rigid deformity, a custom-molded plastic and leather composite lace-up brace (ie, Arizona brace) or a rigid ankle-foot orthosis (AFO) with a molded foot orthosis inside the brace is typically offered. Selective intra-articular corticosteroid injections are also considered in later stages of PTT dysfunction as hindfoot joints become inflamed and arthritic.

OPERATIVE MANAGEMENT

Many combinations of bone and soft tissue procedures have been used in treating AAFD without a clear consensus on an optimal management algorithm.[2,5,11-18] The focus of operative treatment involves restoring PTT function and correcting the resulting deformity. Current practice supports the theory that isolated medial soft tissue procedures only provide temporary functional restoration; therefore, bony corrective procedures of the underlying deformity are necessary to prevent attenuation or failure of the soft tissue repair.[19,20]

Many clinicians think that stage I and II deformities refractory to conservative management can be corrected with PTT debridement, tendon transfer, and a medial displacement calcaneal osteotomy (MDCO). This treatment allows sufficient hindfoot valgus correction to protect the medial soft tissue repair and tendon transfer without sacrificing significant motion.[7,19-23] More significant stage II deformities might require an additional lateral column-lengthening procedure to correct forefoot abduction, or limited joint arthrodeses to optimize correction.[19,23-26] Other clinicians have suggested that subtalar arthroereisis may be advantageous in decreasing the strain on PTT repair and tendon transfer as well.[16] Stage III and IV deformities often require a more extensive arthrodesis procedure in addition to tendon transfers and repairing or reconstructing any deltoid ligament disorder.[27]

Spring ligament and deltoid ligament disorders should be addressed, if present, in the form of direct repair, imbrication, or reconstruction.[4,28,29] It has recently been suggested that AAFD can be caused by an isolated spring ligament injury in the setting of a normal PTT.[30] In these cases, an isolated spring ligament repair may be the only procedure necessary to correct the deformity.[30] If significant forefoot varus remains after initial soft tissue reconstruction and bony procedures, all stages of PTT dysfunction may also require a bony procedure involving the first ray to decrease the risk of excessive loading on the lateral border of the foot and possible deltoid ligament strain,[24] which is often achieved with a Cotton osteotomy,[14,31] reverse Cotton osteotomy,[32] or 1st tarsometatarsal fusion. Triceps surae contractures should also be addressed with a gastrocnemius recession or tendo-Achilles lengthening, because this is a contributing factor in AAFD.[33]

There are many options for reconstruction of AAFD involving both bone and soft tissue work. This article discusses the role of tendon transfers in medial soft tissue restoration in AAFD. Common tendon transfers include flexor digitorum longus (FDL), flexor hallucis longus (FHL), PB in addition to FDL or FHL transfer, and PB to peroneus longus (PL) transfer.

TENDON TRANSFER PRINCIPLES

As recently outlined by Bluman and Dowd,[34] the ideal tendon transfer must possess 5 basic properties to effectively correct deformity and improve motor function.

Thus, donor tendons should have appropriate strength, appropriate excursion, similar direction and attachment as the replaced tendon, a single function, and ideally be in phase with the tendon that it is replacing. Muscle strength (or its ability to generate force) is directly proportional to the cross-sectional area of the muscle, and muscle excursion is directly proportional to fiber length. A 1985 cadaveric study by Silver and colleagues[35] calculated the relative strength and excursion of the muscles about the ankle using these principles. The relative strength of the PTT was 6.4; FHL, 3.6; FDL, 1.8; PL, 5.5; and PB, 2.6. Likewise, the excursion of the PTT was 4.1 cm; FHL, 4.8 cm; FDL, 4.8 cm; PL, 4.7 cm; and PB, 4.1 cm (**Table 2**).

After considering these principles and data, the FHL and FDL seem to be appropriate tendons to replace the diseased PT because they have slightly greater excursions and relative strength that is similar to the antagonistic PB muscle. Both muscles are also in phase with the PT on the medial aspect of the ankle.

DECISIONS INVOLVING THE DISEASED PTT

The first decision in planning for a tendon transfer in AAFD involves managing the diseased PTT. The surgeon must decide whether to debride, excise, or keep the damaged tendon. Aronow[36] discussed the controversy surrounding this topic in a recent review article. He presented theories regarding the diseased PTT: (1) in AAFD, the PTT is a pain generator and pain cannot be alleviated until the tendon is removed; and (2) the PTT is significantly stronger than the muscle tendon units used to replace it, and therefore it should not be sacrificed unnecessarily.

Giving credence to the first theory is the histologic and gross comparisons of patients with stage II dysfunction and presumed normal cadaveric specimens.[37,38] The PTT in affected patients was hypertrophied with loss of normal appearance. Histologic analysis found degenerative tendinosis characterized by increased mucin content, fibroblast hypercellularity, chondroid metaplasia, and neovascularization, which resulted in a markedly disorganized collagen structure. Furthermore, neither acute nor chronic inflammation was identified. In contrast, another publication[37] showed significant fibrosis within the tendon; however, it is unclear whether these changes preceded or postdated PTT dysfunction.

Aronow[36] also indicated that the often-hypertrophied PTT combined with a tendon transfer would be too bulky under a tight flexor retinaculum and possibly would prohibit tendon sheath closure. Therefore, the retained tendon could cause continued discomfort secondary to its bulk or excessive scarring between the tendons and surrounding subcutaneous tissue.

Table 2		
Comparison of tendon properties		
Tendon	**Relative Strength**	**Excursion (cm)**
PTT	6.4	4.1
FDL	1.8	4.8
FHL	3.6	4.8
PB	2.6	4.1
PL	5.5	4.7

Data from Silver RL, de la Garza J, Rang M. The myth of muscle balance. A study of relative strengths and excursions of normal muscles about the foot and ankle. J Bone Joint Surg Br 1985;67:432–7.

Additional evidence that supports excising the diseased PTT includes the resultant hypertrophy and strength gains of the transferred tendon. A study by Rosenfeld and colleagues[39] found that patients who underwent FDL transfer and MDCO for stage II dysfunction had a mean 23% atrophy of the PT muscle and mean 27% hypertrophy of the FDL muscle, as determined by magnetic resonance imaging, compared with the unaffected contralateral side. In patients in whom the PTT was retained, the FDL muscle hypertrophied 11% at 14 months; however, in patients in whom the PTT was excised, the FDL hypertrophied 4 times more to 44% of the contralateral side. This finding suggests that excising the PTT results in a more functional tendon transfer. However, the American Orthopaedic Foot and Ankle Society (AOFAS) hindfoot scores were not significantly different between the retained and excised groups.

Leaving a portion of the PTT intact is supported by the data presented earlier by Silver and colleagues[35] showing that the stronger PT tendon should be preserved if possible to balance the foot against the PB and PL. Aronow[36] recommends that if the distal tendon appears healthy, a repair should be attempted or the tendon transfer should be anastomosed with the distal stump.[36] If the proximal tendon appears healthy and a repair cannot be performed, then the tendon should be tenodesed to the adjacent tendon being transferred.[36]

FDL TRANSFER
Rationale for FDL Transfer

Goldner and colleagues[40] at Duke University were the first to describe FDL and FHL transfer for talipes equinovalgus in 1974. They found that isolated plication of the PTT was insufficient in alleviating pain and restoring the arch. They reported improved results with FDL or FHL transfer in addition to imbrication of the spring ligament and tendo-Achilles lengthening.

The FDL runs anteromedially to the proximal PTT and posterolaterally to the distal PTT without any significant structures in between these two tendons. It can be accessed easily through the same incision used to inspect and debride the PTT, if necessary. Unlike the FHL, the FDL transfer does not require crossing the neurovascular bundle. In addition, as mentioned earlier, the muscle is in phase with the PTT and has similar tendon excursion. Furthermore, if cut proximal to the master knot of Henry, the FDL is partially preserved in many individuals because of FHL and quadratus plantae attachments on the most distal aspect of the tendon. The only disadvantage to an FDL transfer is the weakness of this tendon compared with the antagonistic PB.[35]

FDL Transfer Surgical Technique

Palpation and routine marking of the bony landmarks are necessary in planning any incision on the foot and ankle. This incision extends from just posterior to the medial malleolus to a point just distal to the navicular tuberosity (**Fig. 2**). The flexor retinaculum is left in place and typically not divided. With tenotomy or mayo scissors, dissection is continued and the PTT sheath is identified just posterior to the medial malleolus. The tendon sheath is then sharply divided and the tendon is inspected. Typical gross pathologic findings of the PTT include tenosynovitis, yellowing, thickening, incontinuity or longitudinal tears, and at times a complete tendon rupture (**Fig. 3**).[1,37,38] The tendon is either debrided and repaired or excised based on the surgeon's preference, as discussed earlier. After this is achieved, the toes are flexed and extended to aid in identifying the FDL posterolateral to the distal PTT tendon. The FDL sheath is also divided sharply, exposing the tendon (**Fig. 4**). The ankle is plantarflexed, the hindfoot is supinated, and the lesser toes are flexed to provide as much FDL length as possible

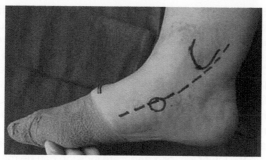

Fig. 2. Typical medial incision for FDL tendon transfer. (*Courtesy of* Jeffrey E. Johnson, MD, Chesterfield, MO.)

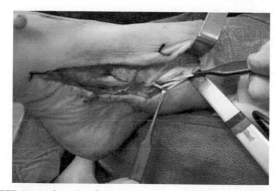

Fig. 3. Ruptured PTT. Note that the flexor retinaculum is left intact posterior to the medial malleolus. (*Courtesy of* Jeffrey E. Johnson, MD, Chesterfield, MO.)

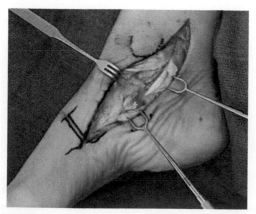

Fig. 4. FDL tendon identified posterior to the medial malleolus after PTT debridement. The tendon was then dissected distally toward the knot of Henry. (*Courtesy of* Jeffrey E. Johnson, MD, Chesterfield, MO.)

during harvest. The tendon is then dissected out distally, elevating the abductor tendon from the plantar-medial aspect of the foot and carefully coagulating the venous plexus that is frequently encountered. Care must also be taken to preserve the medial plantar branch of the tibial nerve, because this structure often lies superficial to the distal FDL. The FDL tendon is then divided sharply just proximal to the master knot of Henry. We think that it is important to take as much tendon as possible to ensure adequate length for transfer. Excess tendon can be trimmed after tensioning. The distal end of the harvested tendon is then controlled with a grasping suture, which aids in manipulating and tensioning the tendon in transfer (**Fig. 5**).

In the event of a ruptured and proximally retracted PTT, the initial incision can be curved proximally up the lower leg, or a separate incision can be made at the myotendinous junction of the PTT and FDL. The proximal PTT stump is debrided and, if an adequate amount appears healthy and the muscle is functional, it can be tenodesed to the proximal FDL tendon, which can be achieved by applying physiologic tension and using a side-to-side repair with braided nonabsorbable suture or a Pulvertaft weave. This step can be performed before or after FDL tendon harvest.

Next, a decision must be made with the portion of FDL that remained in the foot at the point of transection near the knot of Henry. Many clinicians think that losing lesser toe distal interphalangeal strength is not functionally limiting in most patients, because there is some compensation by the quadratus plantae insertion on the distal FDL. Several studies have also shown that there are distal interconnections between the FHL and FDL tendons near the master knot of Henry in most patients.[40–45] Nevertheless, the lesser toes have intact metatarsophalangeal and proximal interphalangeal flexion from the flexor digitorum brevis and the intrinsic muscles of the foot. However, other clinicians think that the distal FDL stump should be tenodesed to the intact FHL (or distal FHL to FDL in an FHL transfer[46,47]) to preserve toe plantarflexion strength.[48]

At this point, the clinician needs to decide where to transfer the FDL tendon. It can be transferred to the intact distal PTT, the ruptured distal PTT stump, or the navicular tuberosity. If the distal PTT is intact, performing a Pulvertaft weave or side-to-side repair recreates the normal biomechanical function of the PT by acting on all of its insertion sites. If the distal PTT is too diseased, or the surgeon prefers to excise it for the reasons mentioned earlier, the FDL can be transferred to the navicular or medial cuneiform. The navicular tuberosity is often chosen, because it requires less FDL

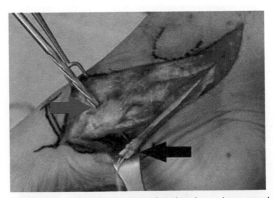

Fig. 5. The black arrow points to the FDL tendon that has been harvested and has a grasping suture in place to aid in transfer. The red arrow points to the drill preparing to create a tunnel through the navicular for FDL transfer. Note that the guide pin exits the plantar aspect of the navicular. (*Courtesy of* Jeffrey E. Johnson, MD, Chesterfield, MO.)

tendon length and inserting the tendon here is thought to provide more powerful hindfoot inversion and forefoot adduction than when inserted into the medial cuneiform. This concept was postulated by Mann,[48] who thought that inserting the tendon on the more medial navicular rather than the medial cuneiform provided an increased moment arm on the subtalar joint axis. This concept was later corroborated by Hui and colleagues[49] in a cadaveric study that reported a 46% decreased moment arm of the FDL when transferred to the navicular as opposed to a 56% decrease when transferred to the medial cuneiform. However, other clinicians argue that transferring the FDL to the medial cuneiform buttresses the plantar medial aspect of the naviculocuneiform joint and prevents the lateral sag often seen with patients who have AAFD.[14]

We prefer to pass the FDL through a bone tunnel in the navicular tuberosity. When making the tunnel, care must be taken to avoid violating any articular surface as well as to maintain an appropriate thickness to the medial wall to avoid breaking the tunnel when the tendon is transferred. The tunnel can be made with a cannulated drill bit over a guide pin to ensure that the trajectory of the tunnel is satisfactory by verifying the location of the guide pin before drilling (see **Fig. 5**; **Fig. 6**). Once the tunnel is created, the FDL is passed from plantar to dorsal. It is tensioned and secured with suture anchors,[50,51] interference screws,[52–55] or by sewing it back on itself (**Fig. 7**). The tendon is transferred and tensioned as the last step in the flatfoot reconstruction after all other bone and soft tissue reconstruction has been completed.

No consensus exists on a technique for achieving ideal tension of the tendon transfer. Hansen[56] placed the foot in slight flexion with hindfoot inversion while tightening the FDL 5 to 10 mm into the medial cuneiform. He then sutured it over the tibialis anterior if possible or the dorsal medial cuneiform capsule. Myerson[57] reported that his team secured the tendon while positioning the foot beyond midline and in inversion.

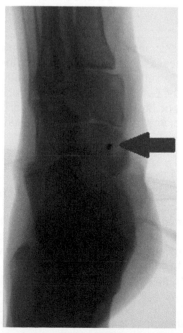

Fig. 6. Intraoperative fluoroscopic image of guide pin (*arrow*) placed in the navicular tuberosity. The drill is used to create a bone tunnel over this guide pin.

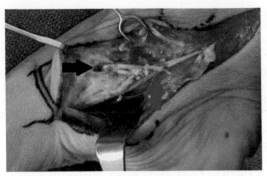

Fig. 7. The FDL tendon has been transferred through the navicular, passed from plantar to dorsal through a bone tunnel (*black arrow*), and then sutured back to itself (*red arrow*). The FDL can also be secured to the periosteum at the dorsal and plantar aspects of the navicular. (*Courtesy of* Jeffrey E. Johnson, MD, Chesterfield, MO.)

He warned that overtightening the FDL and causing it to sublux out of its groove was possible; however, heavy patients and those with a extensive deformity should have tighter repairs. He also argued that the tendon would loosen over time and that the foot would eventually achieve a more neutral position. Haddad and Mann[58] more recently recommend securing the FDL at a midpoint between where the tendon lies in the navicular tunnel in its most relaxed state and at its most tensioned state while adducting the forefoot and inverting the subtalar joint. In conclusion, most investigators recommend securing the tendon with the hindfoot in inversion along with some plantarflexion of the foot. The ideal tension on the tendon seems to be a matter of the personal preference and clinical experience of the surgeon.

FDL Transfer Results

In general, the reports for FDL transfer are favorable in treatment of AAFD; however, it is difficult to isolate the success of the tendon transfer in the setting of so many other concomitant procedures. In an effort to evaluate the effectiveness of FDL transfer, articles that primarily report the outcomes of soft tissue procedures are reviewed here. These reports can generally be broken down into 2 groups: (1) FDL transfer to an intact PTT tendon or distal stump, and (2) FDL transfer to the navicular bone.

FDL transfer to the native distal PTT

In 1982, Jahss[59] described a series of 6 patients who underwent a side-to-side FDL tenodesis proximally and distally to a ruptured PTT. He reported excellent results, with restoration of 20% to 25% of inversion power. In 5 patients in whom a direct repair of a PTT rupture could not be performed, Funk and colleagues[1] described a similar side-to-side proximal and distal FDL transfer to bridge the gap following debridement. At 24 to 32 months' follow-up, all 5 patients could perform a single-limb heel rise and had improvements in subjective pain with weight bearing. Nevertheless, 3 patients continued to complain of mild swelling in the medial hindfoot. Feldman and colleagues[60] described a nearly identical procedure in 11 patients who had stage 2 PTT dysfunction at an average 34 months' follow-up. The mean AOFAS hindfoot score improved from 38.8 to 78.1, and 6 patients reported 90% or greater pain relief.

Shereff[61] reported a series of 17 patients with stage II PTT dysfunction who had debridement and end-to-end repair of the PTT tendon followed by a side-to-side FDL tenodesis. The distal FDL was left intact on its insertion. At 27 months' average follow-up, all patients were able to perform a single-limb heel rise, had 5 out of 5 inversion strength, and all but 1 reported unlimited ambulation. Ten of 17 patients had an arch without weight bearing and 7 had an arch with weight bearing. The AOFAS hindfoot score was improved from an average of 66 before surgery to an average of 96 after surgery and, of the 13 patients who did not have a concurrent subtalar fusion, 11 patients had scores between 80 and 100. The other 2 patients reported fair and poor scores.

However, not all reports are supportive of FDL tenodesis to the native PTT tendon. In 1992, Conti and colleagues[62] noted that 6 of 20 patients who underwent isolated PTT debridement and side-to-side anastomosis of the FDL failed at an average of nearly 15 months. These patients required a triple arthrodesis to relieve their symptoms and restore function. To our knowledge, this is the most negative report of FDL tendon transfers.

FDL transfer to the navicular

Mann and Thompson[63] described a series of 14 patients who underwent an FDL transfer to the navicular and 3 patients with PTT advancement for AAFD. At 2 to 5 years' follow-up, 12 patients had complete pain relief and excellent strength, 1 had complete pain relief with mild weakness (which they attributed to an ankle fracture sustained by the patient after surgery), 3 had some mild persistent pain and weakness, and 1 patient had continued pain despite a functional transfer. The flatfoot deformity was only corrected in 4 patients and 7 had improved arches. The other 6 patients had either no change or worsening of their deformity. Mann[48] later reported that after applying more stringent requirements on deformity flexibility he had less than 5% of more than 100 FDL transfer cases require subsequent fusion at long-term follow-up. His newer criteria consisted of at least 15° of subtalar motion, 10° of talonavicular adduction, and less than 12° of fixed forefoot varus. In contrast, his prior FDL transfer indications resulted in a nearly 90% subsequent fusion rate.

Gazdag and Cracchiolo[4] reported the outcomes of 22 patients who had surgical treatment of stage II PTT dysfunction at an average of 32 months. Eighteen of these patients had spring ligament disorders that required surgery and 17 of these patients required FDL transfer to the navicular as well. Of these 18 patients, 14 had an excellent result, 2 patients had a fair result, and 2 patients had a poor result. Three of the remaining 4 patients without spring ligament disorder also underwent FDL transfer. Two of these patients had excellent results, 1 had a fair result, and 1 had a poor result. The investigators defined an excellent result as those patients who were pain free, able to walk more than 6 blocks, and able to do a single heel rise. Patients with a fair result either did not have complete pain relief or were unable to walk more than 6 blocks, but they were still able to perform a single-limb heel rise. Of the 3 patients with poor results, 1 patient developed complex regional pain syndrome, 1 had continued medial hindfoot pain and was unable to perform a single-limb heel rise, and the last patient had lateral hindfoot pain and an inability to perform a single-limb heel rise in addition to mild talonavicular and subtalar arthritic changes. Radiographic improvement was noted in the 19 patients with excellent and fair results in which the average lateral talo–first metatarsal angle improved from an average of 13° to 9°. The patients with poor results had a decrease in lateral talo–first metatarsal angle from an average of 13° to 20°.

FHL TRANSFER
Rationale for FHL Transfer

As mentioned earlier, the FHL transfer was also described by Goldner and colleagues[40] in their series on treatment of talipes equinovalgus. In their discussion, they noted that the FHL is readily available through a similar incision when assessing the PTT, and that it had a greater muscle mass and more robust tendon compared with the FDL. They also thought that, if the tendon was left underneath the sustentaculum tali, it helped to maintain elevation of the sustentaculum tali and aid in talar reduction following transfer. Silver and colleagues'[35] study validates what Goldner and colleagues[40] found clinically in relation to the tendon size and proportional muscle strength. The FHL tendon is nearly 56% as strong as the tibialis posterior and is almost twice as strong as the FDL; therefore, it provides greater force to counteract the PB.

Nevertheless, many clinicians choose not to use the FHL because it has to be rerouted around the neurovascular bundle and there is concern for functional deficits with decreased hallux plantarflexion strength. Several studies have found that transfer of the FHL for other indications does weaken hallux interphalangeal flexion, but AOFAS Hallux MTP-IP (metatarsophalangeal-interphalangeal) Scale scores remain high[64] and no functional deficits were observed.[65,66] A recent cadaveric study by Spratley and colleagues[47] noted that both FHL and FDL transfer significantly reduced hallux and lesser toe flexion strength; however, when the distal FHL was tenodesed to the FDL, hallux flexion strength was restored almost to pretransfer levels. The FDL transfer with tenodesis also resulted in an increased medial midfoot and heel plantar force compared with FHL transfer and tenodesis. This finding suggests that the FHL may be a more biomechanically appropriate tendon transfer in AAFD treatment; however, further clinical studies are needed to prove this assertion.

FHL Transfer Technique

Using the same medial incision as described earlier, the PTT is exposed and prepared in a similar manner to the FDL transfer procedure. The FHL is identified near the master knot of Henry by flexing and extending the great toe. With the ankle plantarflexed, the hindfoot supinated, and the hallux interphalangeal joint flexed, the FHL tendon is transected just proximal to the master knot of Henry. As described earlier, the distal FHL tendon left at the knot of Henry is either left alone or tenodesed to the FDL tendon, depending on surgeon preference. The FHL tendon is then identified above the flexor retinaculum through an additional proximal incision or the medial incision that is extended proximally. After identification, the tendon is pulled into the proximal aspect of the wound, out of its sheath. A grasping suture is then placed into the distal aspect of the tendon to ease in managing it through transfer. The FHL is then passed deep to the neurovascular bundle, into the PTT sheath, and toward the distal aspect of the wound (**Fig. 8**). A Hewson suture passer or tendon-passing instrument can be helpful in helping to pull the tendon on this course. The FHL tendon is then inserted into the intact distal PTT or ruptured distal PTT stump if it appears healthy. If not, it is inserted into the navicular tuberosity in a similar manner to that described for the FDL tendon. Furthermore, if the proximal PTT is healthy, it can be tenodesed to the proximal FHL in the same manner as the FDL transfer. As with the FDL transfer, the FHL is transferred and fixed with the foot in maximal plantarflexion and inversion, after all other bone and soft tissue procedures in the flatfoot reconstruction have been completed.

FHL Transfer Results

Sammarco and Hockenberry[46] published the largest series of FHL transfers with an MDCO for stage II PTT dysfunction. Seventeen patients were assessed at an average of 18 months' follow-up. The average AOFAS hindfoot score increased from 62.4 to 83.6. Ten patients were satisfied, 6 patients were satisfied with minor reservations, and 1 patient was dissatisfied. No significant improvement was noted clinically or radiographically in the medial longitudinal arch.

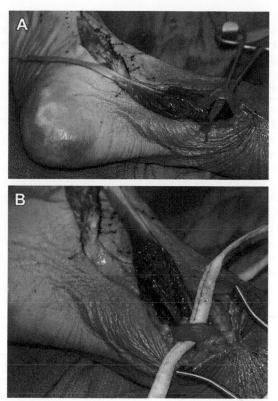

Fig. 8. The FHL tendon is identified and transected at the master knot of Henry. A passing suture is placed into the free end of the tendon. (*A*) The tendon is then brought into the proximal wound at the level of the tibialis posterior myotendinous junction. At this level, the FHL is posteromedial to the neurovascular bundle (protected with a clamp in figure). (*B*) The FHL tendon is passed deep and lateral to the neurovascular bundle. It is then brought distally through the PTT sheath, beneath the flexor retinaculum (see **Fig. 9**B). At this point the tendon is passed through a tunnel in the navicular and secured to itself as previously described for the FDL tendon (see **Fig. 7**). (*From* Aronow MS. Tendon transfer options in managing the adult flexible flatfoot. Foot Ankle Clin 2012;17:205–26.)

Mulier and colleagues[43] studied FHL harvest technique in 24 cadavers through a 2-incision approach and noted 2 complete medial plantar nerve disruptions. They also noted 1 partial disruption of both medial and lateral plantar nerves. Significant nerve stretch was noted in 3 medial plantar nerves and 1 lateral plantar nerve. Therefore, they found a significant risk to the medial and lateral plantar nerves with their FHL harvest technique. The clinical implications of these finding are difficult to interpret in this cadaveric study. However, there is a paucity of literature involving FHL transfer to validate their conclusions.

PB TRANSFER
Rationale for PB Transfer

In 2001, Song and Deland[67] described a supplemental transfer of the PB to the FDL transfer in addition to an MDCO in stage II PTT dysfunction. The senior author added the PB transfer to the FDL tendon transfer in cases in which the FDL tendon was particularly small or had been used previously. They thought that, in addition to removing the principal antagonist to the PTT, the PB tendon would provide additional inversion strength to maintain the medial longitudinal arch. In this article, the PB was transferred in less than 10% of all their patients with AAFD.

PB to FDL Transfer Technique

Using a similar incision to that described for FHL and FDL transfers, the diseased distal PTT is excised after the FDL is tenodesed proximally. The FDL is harvested as described earlier and is transferred into the navicular. An incision is then made at the junction of the glabrous skin near the base of the 5th metatarsal to isolate the PB. It is released from its insertion on the base of the 5th metatarsal and brought out of the skin at a second, more proximal lateral incision above the ankle. A grasping stitch is placed in the end of the tendon to help manipulate the tendon in transfer (**Fig. 9**A). The PB tendon is then passed using a tendon-passing instrument behind the tibia into the proximal medial wound where the proximal FDL to PTT tenodesis was performed (see **Fig. 9**B). The PB tendon is then passed down the PTT sheath and into the same bony navicular tunnel as the FDL. With the foot held in inversion and plantar flexion, both tendons are secured in the bony tunnel using one of the methods described earlier. As with the other transfers, this is performed as the last step in the flatfoot reconstruction, after all other bone and soft tissue procedures have been completed.

PB to FDL Transfer Results

In Song and Deland's[67] series of 13 patients with 20 months' average follow-up, significant weakness was noted in both hindfoot inversion and eversion compared with the contralateral limb; however, only 1 patient had less than 4 out of 5 inversion strength. Compared retrospectively with matched patients who only underwent FDL transfer and an MDCO, no statistical differences were shown in AOFAS hindfoot scores, inversion strength, eversion strength, or range of motion. They concluded that the additional PB tendon transfer is a good option to supplement small FDL tendons or in revision surgery without sacrificing hindfoot eversion strength.

PB to PL Transfer Rationale

Although the PL tendon is antagonistic to the PTT as a powerful hindfoot evertor, it also maintains the medial longitudinal arch by plantarflexing the first ray and supporting the plantar ligaments. Hansen[68] described a PB to PL transfer for young patients with peroneal spastic flatfoot in an effort to exploit the arch-supporting functions of the PL. In a recent review by Aronow,[36] he cited this technique as a possible means to convert a deforming abduction force of the PB to an arch-correcting plantarflexion force on the first metatarsal in patients with AAFD. He also surmised that proximal lengthening of the PB might be beneficial in AAFD by weakening the primary antagonist to the PTT. The risks of these procedures are peroneal tendinopathy, hindfoot eversion weakness, and chronic lateral ankle functional instability; however, these risks have not been proved to occur.[67] Aronow[36] stated that he had not performed any PB-lengthening procedures, but he has performed a PB tenotomy and gastrocnemius recession for a patient with stage III PTT dysfunction undergoing a triple arthrodesis.[36] We have limited experience with PB tenotomy, lengthening, or transfer for patients with AAFD, using it only as a technique to decrease abduction deformity in patients undergoing triple arthrodesis for AAFD. However, no clinical series have been performed to analyze the results of any of these procedures.

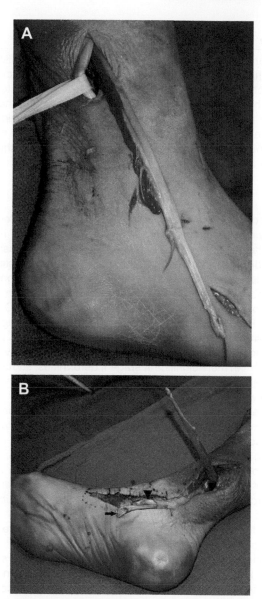

Fig. 9. The PB tendon is harvested through 2 lateral incisions. One is made just proximal to the 5th metatarsal base where the tendon is transected. The second is made just posterior to the fibula, at the level of the PTT myotendinous junction. (*A*) The PB tendon is brought prox- imally through this second incision. A grasping suture is placed through the distal end of the tendon to ease transfer. Using a clamp to aid in tendon transfer, the PB tendon is passed through the proximal incisions from lateral to medial. The transfer is made posterior to the tibia but the PB tendon is kept deep to the PL on the lateral side (*A*), and deep to the medial neurovascular bundle and FHL on the medial side (*B*). The PB tendon is then passed through the PTT sheath into the distal wound and prepared for transfer in a manner previ- ously described for FDL transfer. (*B*) The arrow shows the FHL tendon that was previously transferred in this cadaveric specimen (see **Fig. 8**). The arrowhead shows a completed FDL transfer that was performed in this cadaveric specimen for demonstration. (*From* Aronow MS. Tendon transfer options in managing the adult flexible flatfoot. Foot Ankle Clin 2012;17:205–26.)

PB to PL Technique

As described by Hansen,[68] the PB is transected at the level of the distal calcaneus with the same incision that is used for a lateral column-lengthening procedure. The tendon is allowed to retract 1 to 2 cm and the peroneal sheath and paratenon are removed from the tendon. The PB is tenodesed under minimal tension to the PL by passing it from superficial to deep through a slit in the PL tendon, fastening the tendons to one another with a nonabsorbable suture. As an alternative, the PB may be transected proximal to the superior peroneal retinaculum and tenodesed to the PL under physiologic tension with the foot in a neutral plantigrade position.

SUMMARY

AAFD describes a condition of progressive hindfoot valgus, forefoot abduction, and forefoot varus. It is most commonly caused by PTT dysfunction.[1] Patients who have AAFD often complain of posteromedial hindfoot pain, a progressive change in the shape of the foot, difficulty with weight bearing, and gait abnormalities. Conservative management consists of nonsteroidal antiinflammatory medications, selective corticosteroid injections, and physical therapy. Patients also benefit from temporary immobilization in a cast or boot, custom foot orthosis, or a custom AFO or Arizona brace.

In stage I and II PTT dysfunction, in which conservative management has failed, many clinicians think that the deformity can be corrected with PTT debridement, tendon transfer, and an MDCO.[7,19–23] Spring ligament repair may also be indicated in certain cases.[4,28,29] In more significant stage II deformities, subtalar arthroereisis,[16] an additional lateral column-lengthening osteotomy, and selective fusions may be required.[19,23–26] Few data exist to effectively compare transfers to a retained PTT or distal PTT stump versus transfer into the navicular. The tendon harvested for transfer is based on surgeon preference. FDL[1,4,40,48,59–63] and FHL[40,43,46] transfers have been shown to have good results in AAFD, particularly for stage II PTT dysfunction. There are no comparative studies to differentiate these two procedures; however, the FDL transfer is more commonly used. PB may also be beneficial in supplementing an FDL or FHL transfer in revision cases or patients with small donor tendons.[67] In theory, transfer of the PB to the PL may be beneficial in deformity correction.[36,68] No studies have confirmed the efficacy of this procedure.

At present, most foot and ankle surgeons do not advocate isolated tendon transfers in patients who need correction of AAFD. However, Aronow[36] argued that low-demand elderly patients and young patients with mild to moderate stage II deformities often do well with PTT debridement, spring ligament imbrication or repair, tendon transfer, and a gastrocnemius recession (if necessary) despite incomplete correction of the medial longitudinal arch. He states that the soft tissue procedures can be protected by use of a custom-made supportive orthosis, and, if a limited soft tissue procedure fails, he argues that osteotomies and fusions can be performed at a later date. Although this is reasonable, we caution against isolated soft tissue procedures for correction of AAFD because of the risk of failure and need for further operations.[19,20]

In the case of a stage II flexible flatfoot deformity, our preference is to excise the diseased PTT tendon and use an FDL transfer through a tunnel in the navicular tuberosity. The FDL tendon is typically long enough to pass through the tunnel from plantar to dorsal and be secured back to itself with nonabsorbable suture. The transferred tendon is also sutured to the periosteum of the navicular with nonabsorbable suture at both the plantar and dorsal aspects of the bone tunnel to further secure the tendon. An MDCO is performed in all cases to correct hindfoot valgus deformity. A lateral column-lengthening osteotomy is added when the foot has a significant abduction deformity. A Cotton osteotomy may be required if forefoot varus remains after correcting the hindfoot through calcaneal osteotomies.

Patients with stage III and stage IV deformities typically require a hindfoot arthrodesis.[27] A plantarflexion osteotomy or fusion of the first ray may also be required in patients with persistent forefoot varus.[14,31,32] Furthermore, there may be a role for tendon transfer in patients who undergo hindfoot arthrodesis. Mann and colleagues[69] advocated the addition of an FDL transfer to subtalar arthrodesis to improve the function and deformity in patients with rigid deformities. They thought that the additional tendon transfer would balance the deforming forces created by the PB. It is thought that using an FHL or FDL tendon transfer in the setting of a triple arthrodesis may augment the deformity correction in addition to counteracting the PB.

The decision to proceed with surgical correction of AAFD should be made after conservative treatment options have failed. Careful preoperative planning is necessary to choose the appropriate reconstructive procedures given a patient's clinical examination, deformity, and radiographic findings. Tendon transfers are critical to successful surgical correction of flexible flatfoot deformity and may offer benefit to correction of a more rigid or deformed flatfoot as well.

REFERENCES

1. Funk DA, Cass JR, Johnson KA. Acquired adult flat foot secondary to posterior tibial-tendon pathology. J Bone Joint Surg Am 1986;68:95–102.
2. Pedowitz WJ, Kovatis P. Flatfoot in the adult. J Am Acad Orthop Surg 1995;3: 293–302.
3. Davis WH, Sobel M, DiCarlo EF, et al. Gross, histological, and microvascular anatomy and biomechanical testing of the spring ligament complex. Foot Ankle Int 1996;17:95–102.
4. Gazdag AR, Cracchiolo A 3rd. Rupture of the posterior tibial tendon. Evaluation of injury of the spring ligament and clinical assessment of tendon transfer and ligament repair. J Bone Joint Surg Am 1997;79:675–81.
5. Cohen BE, Ogden F. Medial column procedures in the acquired flatfoot deformity. Foot Ankle Clin 2007;12:287–99, vi.
6. Malicky ES, Crary JL, Houghton MJ, et al. Talocalcaneal and subfibular impingement in symptomatic flatfoot in adults. J Bone Joint Surg Am 2002;84:2005–9.
7. Pinney SJ, Lin SS. Current concept review: acquired adult flatfoot deformity. Foot Ankle Int 2006;27:66–75.
8. Johnson KA, Strom DE. Tibialis posterior tendon dysfunction. Clin Orthop Relat Res 1989;239:196–206.
9. Myerson MS. Adult acquired flatfoot deformity: treatment of dysfunction of the posterior tibial tendon. Instr Course Lect 1997;46:393–405.
10. Alvarez RG, Marini A, Schmitt C, et al. Stage I and II posterior tibial tendon dysfunction treated by a structured nonoperative management protocol: an orthosis and exercise program. Foot Ankle Int 2006;27:2–8.
11. Myerson MS, Corrigan J, Thompson F, et al. Tendon transfer combined with calcaneal osteotomy for treatment of posterior tibial tendon insufficiency: a radiological investigation. Foot Ankle Int 1995;16:712–8.
12. Sands A, Early J, Harrington RM, et al. Effect of variations in calcaneocuboid fusion technique on kinematics of the normal hindfoot. Foot Ankle Int 1998;19: 19–25.
13. Toolan BC, Sangeorzan BJ, Hansen ST Jr. Complex reconstruction for the treatment of dorsolateral peritalar subluxation of the foot. Early results after

distraction arthrodesis of the calcaneocuboid joint in conjunction with stabilization of, and transfer of the flexor digitorum longus tendon to, the midfoot to treat acquired pes planovalgus in adults. J Bone Joint Surg Am 1999;81:1545–60.

14. Hirose CB, Johnson JE. Plantarflexion opening wedge medial cuneiform osteotomy for correction of fixed forefoot varus associated with flatfoot deformity. Foot Ankle Int 2004;25:568–74.

15. Hiller L, Pinney SJ. Surgical treatment of acquired flatfoot deformity: what is the state of practice among academic foot and ankle surgeons in 2002? Foot Ankle Int 2003;24:701–5.

16. Stephens HM, Walling AK, Solmen JD, et al. Subtalar repositional arthrodesis for adult acquired flatfoot. Clin Orthop Relat Res 1999;365:69–73.

17. Habbu R, Holthusen SM, Anderson JG, et al. Operative correction of arch collapse with forefoot deformity: a retrospective analysis of outcomes. Foot Ankle Int 2011;32:764–73.

18. Needleman RL. A surgical approach for flexible flatfeet in adults including a subtalar arthroereisis with the MBA sinus tarsi implant. Foot Ankle Int 2006;27:9–18.

19. Mosier-LaClair S, Pomeroy G, Manoli A 2nd. Operative treatment of the difficult stage 2 adult acquired flatfoot deformity. Foot Ankle Clin 2001;6:95–119.

20. Den Hartog BD. Flexor digitorum longus transfer with medial displacement calcaneal osteotomy. Biomechanical rationale. Foot Ankle Clin 2001;6:67–76, vi.

21. Deland JT. Adult-acquired flatfoot deformity. J Am Acad Orthop Surg 2008;16: 399–406.

22. Myerson MS, Badekas A, Schon LC. Treatment of stage II posterior tibial tendon deficiency with flexor digitorum longus tendon transfer and calcaneal osteotomy. Foot Ankle Int 2004;25:445–50.

23. Guyton GP, Jeng C, Krieger LE, et al. Flexor digitorum longus transfer and medial displacement calcaneal osteotomy for posterior tibial tendon dysfunction: a middle-term clinical follow-up. Foot Ankle Int 2001;22:627–32.

24. Neufeld SK, Myerson MS. Complications of surgical treatments for adult flatfoot deformities. Foot Ankle Clin 2001;6:179–91.

25. Fortin PT. Posterior tibial tendon insufficiency. Isolated fusion of the talonavicular joint. Foot Ankle Clin 2001;6:137–51, vii–viii.

26. Taylor R, Sammarco VJ. Minimizing the role of fusion in the rigid flatfoot. Foot Ankle Clin 2012;17:337–49.

27. Bennett GL, Graham CE, Mauldin DM. Triple arthrodesis in adults. Foot Ankle 1991;12:138–43.

28. Jeng CL, Bluman EM, Myerson MS. Minimally invasive deltoid ligament reconstruction for stage IV flatfoot deformity. Foot Ankle Int 2011;32:21–30.

29. Williams BR, Ellis SJ, Deyer TW, et al. Reconstruction of the spring ligament using a peroneus longus autograft tendon transfer. Foot Ankle Int 2010;31:567–77.

30. Orr JD, Nunley JA 2nd. Isolated spring ligament failure as a cause of adult-acquired flatfoot deformity. Foot Ankle Int 2013;34:818–23.

31. Cotton F. Foot statics and surgery. N Engl J Med 1936;214:353–62.

32. Ling JS, Ross KA, Hannon CP, et al. A plantar closing wedge osteotomy of the medial cuneiform for residual forefoot supination in flatfoot reconstruction. Foot Ankle Int 2013;34(9):1221–6.

33. Van Boerum DH, Sangeorzan BJ. Biomechanics and pathophysiology of flat foot. Foot Ankle Clin 2003;8:419–30.

34. Bluman EM, Dowd T. The basics and science of tendon transfers. Foot Ankle Clin 2011;16:385–99.

35. Silver RL, de la Garza J, Rang M. The myth of muscle balance. A study of relative strengths and excursions of normal muscles about the foot and ankle. J Bone Joint Surg Br 1985;67:432–7.

36. Aronow MS. Tendon transfer options in managing the adult flexible flatfoot. Foot Ankle Clin 2012;17:205–26, vii.

37. Trevino S, Gould N, Korson R. Surgical treatment of stenosing tenosynovitis at the ankle. Foot Ankle 1981;2:37–45.

38. Mosier SM, Lucas DR, Pomeroy G, et al. Pathology of the posterior tibial tendon in posterior tibial tendon insufficiency. Foot Ankle Int 1998;19:520–4.

39. Rosenfeld PF, Dick J, Saxby TS. The response of the flexor digitorum longus and posterior tibial muscles to tendon transfer and calcaneal osteotomy for stage II posterior tibial tendon dysfunction. Foot Ankle Int 2005;26:671–4.

40. Goldner JL, Keats PK, Bassett FH 3rd, et al. Progressive talipes equinovalgus due to trauma or degeneration of the posterior tibial tendon and medial plantar ligaments. Orthop Clin North Am 1974;5:39–51.

41. Oddy MJ, Flowers MJ, Davies MB. Flexor digitorum longus tendon exposure for flatfoot reconstruction: a comparison of two methods in a cadaveric model. Foot Ankle Surg 2010;16:87–90.

42. LaRue BG, Anctil EP. Distal anatomical relationship of the flexor hallucis longus and flexor digitorum longus tendons. Foot Ankle Int 2006;27:528–32.

43. Mulier T, Rummens E, Dereymaeker G. Risk of neurovascular injuries in flexor hallucis longus tendon transfers: an anatomic cadaver study. Foot Ankle Int 2007;28:910–5.

44. O'Sullivan E, Carare-Nnadi R, Greenslade J, et al. Clinical significance of variations in the interconnections between flexor digitorum longus and flexor hallucis longus in the region of the knot of Henry. Clin Anat 2005;18:121–5.

45. Wapner KL, Hecht PJ, Shea JR, et al. Anatomy of second muscular layer of the foot: considerations for tendon selection in transfer for Achilles and posterior tibial tendon reconstruction. Foot Ankle Int 1994;15:420–3.

46. Sammarco GJ, Hockenbury RT. Treatment of stage II posterior tibial tendon dysfunction with flexor hallucis longus transfer and medial displacement calcaneal osteotomy. Foot Ankle Int 2001;22:305–12.

47. Spratley EM, Arnold JM, Owen JR, et al. Plantar forces in flexor hallucis longus versus flexor digitorum longus transfer in adult acquired flatfoot deformity. Foot Ankle Int 2013;34(9):1286–93.

48. Mann RA. Posterior tibial tendon dysfunction. Treatment by flexor digitorum longus transfer. Foot Ankle Clin 2001;6:77–87, vi.

49. Hui HE, Beals TC, Brown NA. Influence of tendon transfer site on moment arms of the flexor digitorum longus muscle. Foot Ankle Int 2007;28:441–7.

50. Myerson MS, Cohen I, Uribe J. An easy way of tensioning and securing a tendon to bone. Foot Ankle Int 2002;23:753–5.

51. Sullivan RJ, Gladwell HA, Aronow MS, et al. An in vitro study comparing the use of suture anchors and drill hole fixation for flexor digitorum longus transfer to the navicular. Foot Ankle Int 2006;27:363–6.

52. Harris NJ, Ven A, Lavalette D. Flexor digitorum longus transfer using an interference screw for stage 2 posterior tibial tendon dysfunction. Foot Ankle Int 2005; 26:781–2.

53. Louden KW, Ambrose CG, Beaty SG, et al. Tendon transfer fixation in the foot and ankle: a biomechanical study evaluating two sizes of pilot holes for bioabsorbable screws. Foot Ankle Int 2003;24:67–72.

54. Sabonghy EP, Wood RM, Ambrose CG, et al. Tendon transfer fixation: comparing a tendon to tendon technique vs. bioabsorbable interference-fit screw fixation. Foot Ankle Int 2003;24:260–2.
55. Wukich DK, Rhim B, Lowery NJ, et al. Biotenodesis screw for fixation of FDL transfer in the treatment of adult acquired flatfoot deformity. Foot Ankle Int 2008;29:730–4.
56. Hansen ST. Transfer of the flexor digitorum communis to the first cuneiform. In: Hansen ST, editor. Functional reconstruction of the foot and ankle. Philadelphia: Lippincott Williams & Wilkins; 2000. p. 430–3.
57. Myerson MS. Correction of flatfoot deformity in the adult. In: Myerson MS, editor. Reconstructive foot and ankle surgery. Philadelphia: Elsevier Saunders; 2005. p. 189–215.
58. Haddad S, Mann RA. Flatfoot in adults. In: Coughlin M, Mann RA, Saltzman C, editors. Surgery of the foot and ankle. St Louis (MO): Mosby; 2011. p. 1007–86.
59. Jahss MH. Spontaneous rupture of the tibialis posterior tendon: clinical findings, tenographic studies, and a new technique of repair. Foot Ankle 1982;3:158–66.
60. Feldman NJ, Oloff LM, Schulhofer SD. In situ tibialis posterior to flexor digitorum longus tendon transfer for tibialis posterior tendon dysfunction: a simplified surgical approach with outcome of 11 patients. J Foot Ankle Surg 2001;40:2–7.
61. Shereff M. Adult flatfoot: posterior tibial tendon dysfunction. Foot Ankle Clin 1997;2:217–361.
62. Conti S, Michelson J, Jahss M. Clinical significance of magnetic resonance imaging in preoperative planning for reconstruction of posterior tibial tendon ruptures. Foot Ankle 1992;13:208–14.
63. Mann RA, Thompson FM. Rupture of the posterior tibial tendon causing flat foot. Surgical treatment. J Bone Joint Surg Am 1985;67:556–61.
64. Richardson DR, Willers J, Cohen BE, et al. Evaluation of the hallux morbidity of single-incision flexor hallucis longus tendon transfer. Foot Ankle Int 2009;30:627–30.
65. Coull R, Flavin R, Stephens MM. Flexor hallucis longus tendon transfer: evaluation of postoperative morbidity. Foot Ankle Int 2003;24:931–4.
66. Den Hartog BD. Flexor hallucis longus transfer for chronic Achilles tendonosis. Foot Ankle Int 2003;24:233–7.
67. Song SJ, Deland JT. Outcome following addition of peroneus brevis tendon transfer to treatment of acquired posterior tibial tendon insufficiency. Foot Ankle Int 2001;22:301–4.
68. Hansen ST. Transfer of the peroneus brevis to the peroneus longus. In: Hansen ST, editor. Functional reconstruction of the foot and ankle. Philadelphia: Lippincott Williams & Wilkins; 2000. p. 439–41.
69. Mann RA, Beaman DN, Horton GA. Isolated subtalar arthrodesis. Foot Ankle Int 1998;19:511–9.

Tendon Transfers in Cavovarus Foot

Cristian Ortiz, MD*, Emilio Wagner, MD

KEYWORDS

- Cavovarus • Foot • Tendon transfers • Charcot-Marie-Tooth

KEY POINTS

- Although not all cavovarus deformities are the same, most of them are related to Charcot-Marie-Tooth disease and are inevitably progressive.
- The challenging cavus foot reconstruction must always include tendon transfers to prevent future deformities, and a careful surgical technique must be used to avoid complications and to increase the success rate.

INTRODUCTION

Cavovarus deformity is defined by fixed equinus of the forefoot on the hindfoot, resulting in a pathologic elevation of the longitudinal arch, with either a fixed or flexible varus hindfoot deformity. The cause is most commonly associated with underlying neurologic disorders, with Charcot-Marie-Tooth disease (or currently known as hereditary sensory motor neuropathy) the most commonly identified diagnosis. This entity is prevalent in approximately 25% of the population and involves a wide spectrum of deformities that require different approaches to correct them. Other neurologic disorders include progressive disorders or lesions, such as myelodysplasia, spinal dysraphism, and syringomyelia.

Classic static neurologic disorders include cerebral palsy and poliomyelitis. These disorders will generate different foot and ankle deformities, depending on which neuromuscular unit is compromised. In this article, the authors focus on the hindfoot and midfoot deformities associated with Charcot-Marie-Tooth disease.

As it has been stated previously in the literature,[1] cavovarus deformity manifests in the growing child with a consequent change in shape and position of bones. The muscle involvement progresses from distal to proximal, affecting primarily the tibialis anterior and peroneus brevis, with secondary dysfunction of the intrinsic muscles. Relative

Disclosure: The authors have no conflicts in relation to the subject or materials discussed in this article.

Orthopedic Department, Clinica Alemana, Vitacura 5951, Vitacura, Santiago, Chile
* Corresponding author.
E-mail address: cortiz@alemana.cl

Foot Ankle Clin N Am 19 (2014) 49–58
http://dx.doi.org/10.1016/j.fcl.2013.10.004 **foot.theclinics.com**

sparing of extensor hallucis longus is observed. This imbalance generates a varus hindfoot as the posterior tibialis remains unopposed by the peroneus brevis, creating a varus moment. The relative weakness of the anterior tibialis relative to the peroneus longus results in plantar flexion of the first metatarsal, which results in midfoot supination, and contributes to a forefoot-driven hindfoot varus. Secondary to weakness of the anterior tibialis muscle, recruitment of extensor hallucis longus occurs, resulting in a cock-up deformity of the great toe, with further depression of the metatarsal head and plantar contracture.

As a general principle, the imbalance must be corrected by canceling the deforming forces and improving the deficit; this is when tendon transfers become necessary. It has been reported that in cases when tendon transfers were not performed, the recurrence rate was higher.[2] Performing arthrodesis in the foot does not preclude the need of adding tendon transfers because a correctly performed fusion may deform over time from an imbalance in the remaining motion segments and result in the recurrence of the deformity.[3]

CLINICAL EXAMINATION

In our examination, we must be able to establish all levels of imbalance present in the cavovarus deformity. A detailed history will reveal episodes of ankle instability or a giving-way sensation, difficulty with uneven surfaces, an awkward gait explained by a mild drop foot, and an inability to use normal shoes because of the common injuries sustained when performing common daily activities, such as walking. Patients should be examined while seated and facing the examiner; the examination should also include standing and walking. A common and evident finding on the physical examination is the peek-a-boo heel sign described by Manoli and Graham.[4] This sign is present when one can see the medial aspect of the heel from the front, as can be seen in **Fig. 1**. This sign is not present when there is a valgus or neutral hindfoot position. Some other findings are hindfoot varus, claw toes, and an elevated arch. The presence of calf atrophy should be observed as well as a drop foot and altered balance while walking. The range of motion of every hindfoot and midfoot joint should be evaluated, assessing the flexibility or stiffness of the deformity and the deforming forces. Flexibility of the hindfoot should be tested by the Coleman block test. In this test, a 1-in

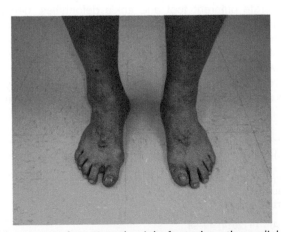

Fig. 1. Patient with cavovarus foot. Note the right foot where the medial side of the heel is noticeable much easier than the left side. This clinical sign is called *peek-a-boo*.

block is placed under the lateral side of the foot, allowing the first metatarsal bone to drop. If the hindfoot is flexible and the hindfoot varus position is completely driven by a pronated forefoot, one will observe correction of the heel varus into valgus. If the heel alignment does not correct, a hindfoot fixed varus will be determined; a surgical procedure must address this deformity.[1] The excursion and strength of the extensors and flexors of the ankle and foot have to be measured and graded because this information combined with the joint range of motion will give us the clue for which muscles represent deforming forces and, thus, should be transferred and which muscles are deficient and, thus, should be augmented with transfers. Soft tissue contractures must be evaluated too. Achilles tendon contracture must be evaluated with the Silfverskiold test. If positive (inability to dorsiflex past 90° is observed with extension of the knee), a gastrocnemius contracture is diagnosed; it should be treated with a proximal gastrocnemius recession. If an equinus contracture is seen throughout the complete knee range of motion, then a formal Achilles tendon lengthening is indicated. The forefoot must be examined for toe deformities, including claw hallux, claw toes, callus, and pain under the metatarsal heads.

GENERAL CONSIDERATIONS FOR TENDON TRANSFERS

The general principles for tendon transfers are listed in **Box 1**. It was Mayer[5] who described many of the principles of tendon transfers still in use today. Although these principles are still valid, some additional details have been incorporated over time[6] but are not the focus of this article.

Stable attachment of the tendon to bone is requisite for the long-term proper functioning of a tendon transfer. Different techniques have been described, including pull out using a button to fix the tendon, weaving the tendon through the bone, anchors, and the newer and most commonly used interference screw techniques. Tension should correspond to half of the tendon excursion; although if there is any doubt, the authors prefer to leave it with a little bit more tension.

These ideal criteria are not always fully present; however, that should not impede us from performing the tendon transfer because we will eliminate a deforming force and support a deficient tendon action.

Tendon transfers should be performed after fixed deformities are corrected to achieve the appropriate tension of the tendon transferred. Some controversy remains as to whether performing tendon transfers and osteotomies early avoids triple arthrodesis in the future.[7] As a general rule, the authors prefer to indicate surgery as soon as patients begin with symptoms unresponsive to medical treatment. Good results can be expected after correction of cavovarus deformity at the long-term follow-up after static and dynamic deformities are corrected.[2]

Box 1
General requirements for tendon transfers

1. The tendon to be transferred should have similar strength (at least grade 4).

2. The tendon should be inserted close to the tendon to be replaced and routed without angulation.

3. There should be flexibility of the joints involved with the tendon transfer.

4. Fixation of the tendon should be to the bone directly or indirectly using another tendon.

5. Agonists are preferable to antagonists.

TREATMENT STRATEGY

The authors plan their surgical decisions based on the level of deformity, which musculotendinous unit represent the deforming forces, and which need supplementation. The authors propose the surgical strategy in **Fig. 2** after the static deformities have been addressed.[1] Incisions must be planned carefully, especially when several incisions and osteotomies are performed at the same time.

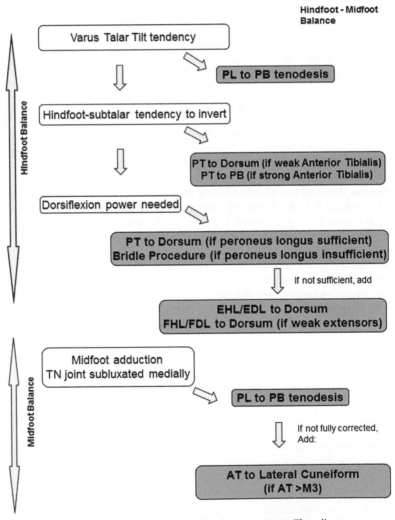

Fig. 2. Treatment strategy for tendon transfers in cavovarus. The diagram presents the problem to treat or consider in white boxes and the surgical procedure in gray boxes. Different options are included relative to the hindfoot first and then the midfoot. AT, anterior tibialis tendon; EDL, extensor digitorum longus; EH, extensor hallucis longus; PB, peroneus brevis tendon; PL, peroneus longus tendon; PT, posterior tibial tendon; TN, talonavicular joint.

PERONEUS LONGUS TO BREVIS TRANSFER

The most commonly performed tendon transfer is the peroneus longus to brevis to decrease the plantar flexion force of the peroneus longus and to increase the eversion power of the brevis to correct flexible varus. The maximal advantage is achieved in younger patients. In the authors' protocol of treatment, it is the most common transfer performed; generally, it is indicated for ankle varus and/or ankle instability.[8] The transfer can be done proximally behind the distal fibula, in the retromalleolar region through a 2-cm incision (**Fig. 3**), or distal to the fibula (**Fig. 4**). The surgical options include using the same incision for the osteotomy of the calcaneus or through an incision close to the peroneus brevis incision at the base of the fifth metatarsal. The peroneus longus is pulled distally under maximal tension and then slightly released to be sutured to the brevis. The suture can be performed with a pulvertaft weave or in a side-to-side fashion.

The authors prefer the retromalleolar approach because it is the easiest and safest in their hands. After cutting the peroneus longus and pulling it distally as far as possible, the authors release the tension slightly and suture it side by side to the peroneus brevis, holding the ankle in neutral flexion and eversion. The authors prefer to use a nonabsorbable suture, with at least 8 connection points between each tendon, preferably with a running-locked suture, which can withstand forces well beyond physiologic loads.

POSTERIOR TIBIAL TENDON TRANSFER TO THE CUNEIFORMS

Following the authors' surgical strategy, the tendency to invert and the dorsiflexion power are evaluated. Most of the authors' patients present with a weak anterior tibialis tendon. The peroneus longus to brevis tendon will help stabilize the ankle[8] but will not be enough to stabilize the hindfoot. Therefore, the second most common tendon transfer that the authors perform is tibialis posterior to one of the cuneiform bones. This transfer eliminates the principal deforming force of the hindfoot, which is the posterior tibialis, and reinforces the weak anterior tibialis. The chosen cuneiform depends on where the deformity is best corrected, and there is no general rule for all cases. This transfer is particularly necessary in Charcot-Marie-Tooth disease. It must be remembered that even a weak posterior tibial tendon should be transferred

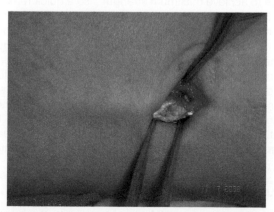

Fig. 3. Clinical picture of peroneus longus to brevis tenodesis. Right foot, inframalleolar region, just proximal to base of the fifth metatarsal bone. Through a small 2-cm-long incision, the peroneus longus is sutured side by side to the peroneus brevis tendon.

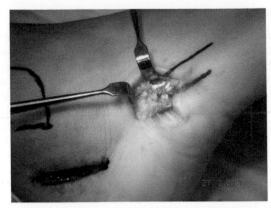

Fig. 4. Clinical picture of right foot, lateral side on the supramalleolar region. A side-to-side tenodesis was performed between the peroneus longus and brevis tendon through a small 1.5-cm-long incision.

because the deforming force is canceled and at least a tenodesis effect will be obtained to aid dorsiflexion.[3] In order to obtain optimal function from the transfer, the contracted posterior soft tissues must be released or lengthened. Most of the time, the posterior tibial tendon is just long enough to be transferred to the cuneiforms; therefore, a careful surgical technique must be used to obtain as much tendon as possible. If the tendon length is inadequate, a turndown flap can be performed or a formal graft can be used[9] (the latter is rarely necessary).

The author's preferred technique is to perform the transfer through the interosseous membrane, harvesting the tendon as distal as possible from a medial incision over the navicular bone. It is then passed proximally to an incision placed medially over the leg, 15 cm above the ankle joint. A third incision is performed over the anterior tibia, 12 cm above the ankle joint line; the tendon is retrieved through the interosseous membrane, taking care in opening a wide window in the interosseous membrane with the help of long scissors or right-angle clamps. From this point, the tendon is passed subcutaneously to the dorsum of the foot where a fourth incision is placed over the cuneiforms. Considering the length of the harvested tendon, interference screw fixation has been the authors' choice to achieve maximum strength[10] so a quick rehabilitation protocol can be used (**Fig. 5**). It has been shown that early active motion is preferable and can decrease the rehabilitation time.[11] To achieve a correct tendon tension, the authors do not use anchors or the self-tensioning technique described for the interference screw because it has been difficult and unreliable in obtaining the appropriate tendon tension. It is the authors' preference to perform a transosseous tensioning technique. This technique is done by perforating the bone when drilling for the screw placement and then using a needle to pass to the plantar aspect of the foot. The needle holds a suture attached to the tendon; thus, tension is applied as wished from the plantar aspect of the foot, pulling the tendon into the tunnel previously created and leaving it with the tension the surgeon prefers. It is then fixed with the interference screw (**Fig. 6**).

POSTERIOR TIBIALIS TO PERONEUS BREVIS TRANSFER

Although this transfer is seldom used, it is considered when the cavovarus foot deformity presents with a strong anterior tibialis; thus, the deformity mainly consists in of an adductovarus without a loss in dorsiflexion strength.[3] For this transfer, the posterior

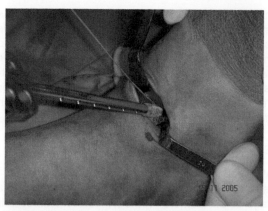

Fig. 5. Right foot, dorsal aspect. When performing a posterior tibial to cuneiform transfer, a biotenodesis screw is used but as an interference screw, pulling the transferred tendon from the plantar aspect of the foot in order to obtain optimal tension.

tibial tendon harvest is performed as already described, and then it is passed deep to the deep posterior muscle compartment of the leg and recovered through the lateral retromalleolar incision previously described for the peroneus longus to brevis tenodesis. At this point, it is sutured side by side to the peroneus brevis.

BRIDLE PROCEDURE

The bridle procedure has been described by Rodriguez[12] and is particularly useful when there is a severe peroneal muscular deficit. It consists of transferring the posterior tibial tendon and adding the peroneus longus and tibialis anterior. The posterior tibial tendon is passed through the tibialis anterior after passing through the interosseous membrane (similar to posterior tibialis to cuneiform transfer). Then the peroneus longus is harvested by a lateral incision over the peroneal tendons, cutting it as proximal as possible and retrieving it through a distal approach just proximal to the base of the fifth metatarsal. It is then transferred subcutaneously from lateral to anterior and

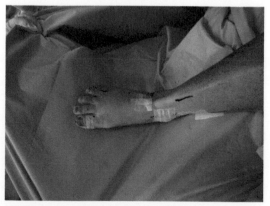

Fig. 6. Dorsal view of a reconstructed foot with a posterior tibial to lateral cuneiform transfer. The transfer is situated in the most appropriate axis to control inversion and eversion. Additional hallux valgus interphalangeus was treated at the same time, explaining the soft dressing over the hallux.

retrieved through the anterior incision where the posterior tibialis was passed through the anterior tibialis. In this area, the peroneus longus is sutured in adequate tension to the anterior tibialis in order to obtain a properly well-balanced midfoot (**Figs. 7** and **8**). Finally, the posterior tibial tendon is secured onto the lateral cuneiform. The authors have obtained a better balanced foot when the anterior tibialis and the peroneus longus tendons are sutured to the posterior tibial tendon. With the appropriate tension added with these tenodeses, an inversion and eversion control is achieved, thus, producing a bridle effect.

TENDON TRANSFERS TO AID IN DORSIFLEXION POWER

When the hindfoot inversion tendency has already been corrected, the next issue to correct is the loss of active dorsiflexion power. This loss should have already been treated at this stage in the authors' strategy, but sometimes additional transfers have to be performed to reinforce the action of the posterior tibialis transfer in allowing active dorsiflexion of the ankle. This surgical decision has to be made preoperatively when the posterior tibialis is a weak muscle (less than grade 3) or when performing revision surgery if a previous transfer has failed in achieving active dorsiflexion. In these cases, the in-phase transfers that can be added are the extensor hallucis longus or the extensor digitorum longus to the dorsal midfoot.[3] These tendons are harvested in the dorsum over the midfoot and secured over the cuneiforms through bone tunnels using biotenodesis screws. The second option is using out-of-phase transfers, which can be used if the extensors previously mentioned are weak or if the dorsiflexion loss is the main symptom and the posterior tibialis transfer has already been made. These transfers are more commonly used in spastic equinovarus deformities. Out-of-phase transfers include the flexor hallucis longus and the flexor digitorum longus tendon,[9] which can be transferred as one unit or isolated. They are transferred through the interosseous membrane and sutured to the anterior tibialis or fixed to the cuneiform bones.

ANTERIOR TIBIALIS TO CUNEIFORMS

This transfer is mainly used after the hindfoot has been corrected and residual midfoot supination is present. The anterior tibialis is generally weak, but it can be part of the

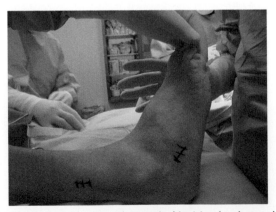

Fig. 7. Lateral view of a right foot where the surgical incision has been planned for a bridle procedure. The peroneus longus tendon is identified through the proximal incision, cut proximally, and then recovered through the distal incision. Then it is passed subcutaneously to the anterior aspect of the ankle joint.

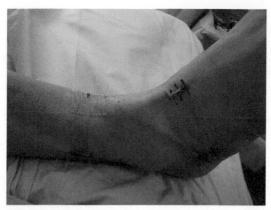

Fig. 8. Same patient from **Fig. 7**. Bridle procedure is complete; the incision over the middle cuneiform is visible where the posterior tibial tendon was fixed. Note the prominence produced by the peroneus longus tendon when traveling from the base of the fifth metatarsal bone to the anterior aspect of the ankle.

deforming forces present that contribute to midfoot supination. Whenever the midfoot or hindfoot remains unbalanced after the transfers already mentioned and the anterior tibialis presents with a relative force of grade 3 or greater, consideration can be given to this transfer.[13]

A medial incision over the anterior tibialis insertion on the medial cuneiform is performed. The tendon is harvested and tubularized at its end and retrieved proximal to the extensor retinaculum. The tendon is then transferred to the dorsum of the foot subcutaneously onto the middle or lateral cuneiform or even the cuboid bone. In this position, it is fixed with a biotenodesis screw with a similar technique as previously described.

POSTOPERATIVE MANAGEMENT

Although the authors authorize full weight bearing as tolerated from the beginning, they keep a removable boot for 6 to 8 weeks to walk and at least for 3 months to sleep at night. Passive movements are instructed after removing the stitches at 2 weeks, and active passive exercises are started at 4 weeks. Physical therapy is initiated at 1 month, stimulating walking with full weight bearing as tolerated, aerobic exercises without impact, and proprioceptive exercises.

SUMMARY

Although not all cavovarus deformities are the same, most of them are related to Charcot-Marie-Tooth disease and inevitably progressive. The challenging cavus foot reconstruction must always include tendon transfers to prevent future deformities, and a careful surgical technique must be used to avoid complications and to increase the success rate.

REFERENCES

1. Ortiz C, Wagner E, Keller A. Cavovarus foot reconstruction. Foot Ankle Clin 2009; 14(3):471–87.

2. Ward CM, Dolan LA, Bennett DL, et al. Long-term results of reconstruction for treatment of a flexible cavovarus foot in Charcot-Marie-Tooth disease. J Bone Joint Surg Am 2008;90:2631–42.
3. Ryssman DB, Myerson MS. Tendon transfers for the adult flexible cavovarus foot. Foot Ankle Clin 2011;16:435–50.
4. Manoli AM, Graham B. The subtle cavus foot, the under pronator, a review. Foot Ankle Int 2005;26(3):256–63.
5. Mayer L. The physiologic method of tendon transplantation. I. Historical, anatomy and physiology of tendons. Surg Gynecol Obstet 1916;22:182–97.
6. Bluman EM, Dowd T. The basics and science of tendon transfers. Foot Ankle Clin 2011;16:385–99.
7. Krause F, Wing K, Alastair Y. Neuromuscular issues in cavovarus foot. Foot Ankle Clin 2008;13:243–58.
8. Vienne P, Schöniger R, Helmy N, et al. Hindfoot instability in cavovarus deformity: static and dynamic balancing. Foot Ankle Int 2007;28(1):96–102.
9. Bibbo C, Jaglan SS. Tendon transfers for equinovarus deformity in adults and children. Foot Ankle Clin 2011;16:401–18.
10. Núñez-Pereira S, Pacha-Vicente D, Llusá-Pérez M, et al. Tendon transfer fixation in the foot and ankle: a biomechanical study. Foot Ankle Int 2009;30(12):1207–11.
11. Rath S, Schreuders T, Stam H, et al. Early active motion versus immobilization after tendon transfer for foot drop deformity. A randomized clinical trial. Clin Orthop Relat Res 2010;468:2477–84.
12. Rodriguez RP. The bridle procedure in the treatment of paralysis of the foot. Foot Ankle Int 1992;13:63–9.
13. Krause F, Henning J, Pfander G, et al. Cavovarus foot realignment to treat antero-medial ankle arthrosis. Foot Ankle Int 2013;34:54–64.

may help determine the etiology. The overall neurovascular status of the limbs is of great importance, especially if surgery is considered.

Radiographic evaluation is usually performed after completing clinical examination. Weight-bearing images of the foot and ankle are carefully assessed to further evaluate the deformity and look for other deformities, possible causes, and underlying arthritis or subluxation of joints (**Fig. 2**). It is essential in evaluating deformities of the foot and ankle to obtain weight-bearing views, because it may accentuate any deformity. Other imaging modalities or nerve conduction studies may be required depending on the suspected etiology.

Treatment

Conservative treatment should be attempted initially. Footwear with a wide, tall toe box to alleviate any impingement on the toes is advocated. Flat heels are encouraged, and shoes with soft padding can be tried. High heels should be abandoned, because they increase the load transferred to the forefoot. Taping and strapping may be useful in flexible deformities but do not provide a permanent solution. Nonsteroidal anti-inflammatory drugs (NSAIDs) may be used for analgesia. An intra-articular corticosteroid injection may improve associated synovitis but does not address the deformity and carries the risk of iatrogenic tendon or capsular disruption.

The role of the FHL, EHL, and PL as etiologic factors for clawed hallux has already been proven in many studies and is believed to present the underlying rationale for current treatment strategies. Procedures utilizing the EHL, namely the Jones and modified Jones procedures, remain the most commonly used operative procedures for hallux claw toe. It was originally described by Jones[8] in 1916. It entails transfer of the EHL into the neck of the first metatarsal. Development of flexion deformity as a complication to some cases led to the evolution of the modified Jones procedure, which consisted of fusion of IP joint in addition to the EHL tendon transfer.

Jones procedure

A medial incision is made along the hallux MTP joint and carried distally into the IP joint. The tendon of the EHL is carefully dissected, then cut 1 cm from its insertion into the IP joint. A drill hole is made into the inferomedial aspect of the first metatarsal neck and continued to the dorsolateral aspect of the metatarsal neck. The tendon is passed through the tunnel, then sutured to itself and to the periosteum. Fusion of the IP joint is then performed after preparation of the joint, typically with a cancellous screw.

Despite having successful results, the modified Jones procedure is associated with multiple drawbacks. Breusch and colleagues[9] found that 48 of 81 patients complained of postoperative catching of the hallux, while 21 of 81 patients displayed transfer

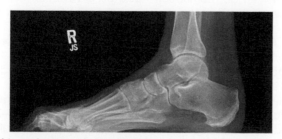

Fig. 2. Radiographic evaluation of claw hallux.

metatarsalgia. Other potential complications include nonunion of the IP joint and other transfer problems.

The authors also transferred the PL to the peroneus brevis in concurrence with the modified Jones procedure and found encouraging patient satisfaction rates. Hansen and colleagues[10] reported patient dissatisfaction with the modified Jones procedure from the lack of toe dorsiflexion and consequent stiffness. In correspondence, he proposed transferring the FHL from the distal phalanx to the base of the proximal phalanx, eliminating the need for IP fusion and maintaining the tendon of the EHL.

FHL transfer technique

A medial midline incision is performed along the hallux MTP joint extending to the IP joint. The sheath of the FHL is identified and incised after proper identification and retraction of the medial neurovascular bundle. The FHL tendon is then cut at its most distal attachment to the distal phalanx. A midline hole is then drilled into the proximal phalanx about 1 cm distal to the joint. The tendon is then passed through the hole from plantar to dorsal. After adequate tensioning until the toe is in a neutral position, the tendon is then resutured to itself and the periosteum along the medial side of the proximal phalanx.

A study by Kadel and colleagues[11] evaluated the role of FHL transfer as an alternative to the modified Jones procedure. They reported on 19 patients (22 FHL transfers). Thirteen (68%) patients reported complete satisfaction; 6 (32%) patients were somewhat satisfied, while none reported dissatisfaction. However, all their patients received concomitant procedures, which might interfere with the interpretation of their results. Another study compared the modified Jones procedure with FHL transfer in a cadaver model and found that they both were equally effective in correcting the angular deformities at the MTP and IP joints as well as reducing the plantar pressure underneath the metatarsal head.

SUMMARY

Claw hallux is a deformity of the great toe attributed to muscular imbalance of various structures. Careful physical examination is important to understand the deforming forces. Various conservative treatments should be employed before surgery is considered. The modified Jones technique is an effective procedure for correcting deformity.

REFERENCES

1. Dwyer FC. The present status of the problem of pes cavus. Clin Orthop 1975;106: 254–75.
2. Lambrinudi C. The feet of the industrial worker: functional aspect: action of the foot muscles. Lancet 1938;2:1480.
3. Paulos L, Coleman SS, Samuelson KM. Pes cavovarus: review of a surgical approach using selective soft-tissue procedures. J Bone Joint Surg Am 1980; 62-A:42–53.
4. Saunders JT. Etiology and treatment of claw foot: report of the results in one hundred and two feet treated by anterior torsal resection. Arch Surg 1935;30:179–98.
5. Faraj AA. Modified Jones procedure for post-polio claw hallux deformity. J Foot Ankle Surg 1997;36(5):356–9.
6. Giannini S, Girolammi M, Ceccarelli F, et al. Modified Jones operation in the treatment of pes cavovarus. Ital J Orthop Traumatol 1985;11(2):165–70.
7. Olson SL, Ledoux WR, Ching RP, et al. Muscular imbalances resulting in a clawed hallux. Foot Ankle Int 2003;24:477–85.

8. Jones R. The soldier's foot and the treatment of common deformities of the foot. Br Med J 1916;1:749–52.

9. Breusch SJ, Wenz W, Doderlein L. Function after correction of a clawed great toe by a modified Robert Jones transfer. J Bone Joint Surg Br 2000;82-B(2):250–4.

10. Hansen ST. Functional reconstruction of the foot and ankle. Philadelphia: Lippincott Williams & Wilkins; 2000.

11. Kadel NJ, Donaldson-Fletcher EA, Hansen ST, et al. Alternative to the modified jones procedure: outcomes of the flexor hallucis longus (FHL) tendon transfer procedure for correction of clawed hallux. Foot Ankle Int 2005 Dec;26(12): 1021–6.

Tendon Transfers for the Drop Foot

Karl M. Schweitzer Jr, MD, Carroll P. Jones, MD*

KEYWORDS

- Tendon transfers • Drop foot • Posterior tibial tendon transfer • Bridle procedure

KEY POINTS

- The paralytic drop foot represents a challenging problem for even the most experienced orthopedic surgeon.
- Careful patient selection, thorough preoperative examination and planning, and application of tendon transfer biomechanical and physiologic principles outlined here can lead to successful results, either through a PT tendon transfer, Bridle transfer, or variations on these procedures.
- Achilles lengthening or gastrocnemius recession may also be needed at the time of tendon transfer.

INTRODUCTION

Tendon transfers are used around the ankle to recreate a balanced foot that is plantigrade and functional.[1,2] Historically, patients with poliomyelitis benefitted from the development and application of tendon transfers throughout the lower extremity, particularly within the foot and ankle to restore strength, balance, and function to a paralytic foot. Although this disease has been essentially eradicated through vaccination, foot and ankle surgeons commonly use tendon transfers for the paralytic foot for other etiologies. The indications are generally divided into four categories: (1) cavovarus, (2) equinovarus, (3) flail, and (4) the topic of this article, drop foot.[3]

In its most basic form, drop foot is defined as the failure of active foot dorsiflexion, which is the end result of a variety of processes. The cause may be neurologic, systemic, or traumatic.[3,4] The neurologic causes are categorized as either central or peripheral. Central neurologic causes include lumbar spinal pathology, closed head injuries, stroke, and multiple sclerosis. Peripheral processes to consider include peroneal nerve palsy; compartment syndrome; and neuropathies, such as Charcot-Marie-Tooth disease.[3]

OrthoCarolina, Charlotte, NC, USA
* Corresponding author. OrthoCarolina, Foot and Ankle Institute, 2001 Vail Avenue, Suite 300, Charlotte, NC 28207.
E-mail address: carroll.jones@orthocarolina.com

Foot Ankle Clin N Am 19 (2014) 65–71
http://dx.doi.org/10.1016/j.fcl.2013.12.002
1083-7515/14/$ – see front matter © 2014 Elsevier Inc. All rights reserved.

foot.theclinics.com

Depending on the cause and severity of the drop foot, the initial recommended conservative treatments consist of Achilles stretching, muscular rehabilitation, and bracing. The most effective brace to address drop foot is an ankle-foot orthosis (AFO). Surgery may be the best initial care if there is an identifiable and treatable central or peripheral nerve problem that could result in motor recovery (ie, lumbar nerve root decompression). For cases of drop foot that are at least a year old with little chance of motor improvement, a tendon transfer may be considered to provide active dorsiflexion.[1–4]

Drop foot is not necessarily just a result of dorsiflexion weakness. There may be associated soft tissue contractures and arthrofibrosis.[4] Failure to recognize all of the contributing factors can lead to inadequate correction and failure of treatment. Patient-specific factors that are also important to consider include expectations and their mental and physical abilities to participate in the crucial postoperative period. In some cases, treatment of a drop foot with an AFO may be the more reasonable option.[3,4]

Goldner's[5] approach to the paralytic foot involved identification of the primary cause or lesion, assessment of the mobility of the foot, vascular examination, sensory evaluation, strength testing of all relevant musculotendinous units, and patient-specific factors. This basic algorithm is essential to assembling a comprehensive, realistic, and effective treatment plan for each patient.

TENDON TRANSFER BASICS

Reports of tendon transfers are found in the literature as early as 1881. Mayer[6] outlined five fundamental tenets of tendon transfer in 1937. These included restoration of the anatomic relationship between a tendon and its sheath, tendon routing through tissue that allows for proper gliding, restoration of normal tendon tension, recreating the anatomic tendon insertion, and establishing proper line of tendon pull.

Musculotendinous units are defined by the gait cycle phase in which they are active. In general, in-phase transfers function most efficiently and effectively.[1,7,8] Although at the time the only option available, out-of-phase transfers are less ideal because of greater muscle strength loss and the need for greater muscle retraining.[2] Out-of-phase transfers are thought to function as static restraints to deformity (ie, tenodesis), not truly undergoing phase conversion, as previously suspected.[1,8,9]

Jeng and Myerson[2] outline several essential points to consider when planning tendon transfers. The function of a tendon is determined by its position relative to the joint under consideration (ie, tendons that run posterior to the ankle and medial to the subtalar joint function as plantarflexors and invertors) and the distance from the tendon to the joint axis, because this determines the effective lever arm for force application across a joint. Musculotendinous units form antagonist force couples (ie, posterior tibialis [PT] and peroneus brevis tendons). Loss of one component of this force couple leads to deformity dictated by its antagonist.

The relative strengths of the tendons involved determine the magnitude of this force differential. Silver and colleagues[10] determined these relative strength values for muscles acting on the foot and ankle and demonstrated a greater degree of complexity than previously suspected. The sum of the relative strength units for the dorsiflexors did not equal that for the plantarflexors (9.4 vs 69 strength units, respectively), and similarly for the evertors and invertors (11.9 and 60.9 strength units, respectively), suggesting a complex level of modulation through the central nervous system (CNS) in balancing these antagonistic forces.[1] These large differentials are realized in CNS injuries (ie, stroke, traumatic brain injury, cerebral palsy), for example, with the development of an equinovarus deformity caused by relative overpull by the plantarflexors and invertors of the ankle and hindfoot.

Consideration should be given to establishing the appropriate amount of tension in the transferred tendon. From Blix curve it is known that fixing a tendon at maximal length creates a tenodesis-effect, versus an ineffective force generator at its most relaxed position.[11] Thus, it is generally preferred to set the tendon tension midway between these two positions to generate the most effective pull.

PT TENDON TRANSFER FOR DROP FOOT: HISTORICAL PERSPECTIVE AND RESULTS

Transfer of the PT tendon to the dorsal foot is well described in the literature for treatment of drop foot.[6,12–20] Wagenaar and Louwerens[21] provide a comprehensive historical summary (see Table IV in Ref.[21]) of the spectrum of results of PT tendon transfer for drop foot. Mayer[6] was the first to describe its use in patients with traumatic paralytic peroneal palsy. Watkins and colleagues[13] described their technique of PT tendon transfer anteriorly through the interosseous membrane to restore dorsiflexion of the foot and reported on 29 patients who underwent the procedure. Lipscomb and Sanchez[15] reported good results in 9 of 10 patients undergoing PT tendon transfer along with triple hindfoot arthrodesis for common peroneal nerve palsy. Turner and Cooper,[18] in their report on 36 patients, found that only 3 out of 15 patients obtained satisfactory results when the PT transfer was used to provide active dorsiflexion of the foot. Several modifications and improvements have been made to these original techniques and are reviewed in the sections that follow.

TENDON TRANSFER PROCEDURES FOR DROP FOOT: PERONEAL NERVE PALSY

For peroneal neuropathy primarily affecting the anterior compartment musculature, the PT tendon is generally transferred through the interosseous membrane to the middle cuneiform by interference screw tendon-bone fixation to restore ankle dorsiflexion.[1–4] In the presence of concomitant peroneal tendon weakness or palsy, PT tendon transfer to the lateral cuneiform is recommended to balance the unopposed inversion pull of the remaining medial toe flexors.[3] If tendon-bone interference fixation is compromised (ie, in case of poor bone stock), then consideration can be given to supplemental fixation using a suture button tied over a bolster to the plantar foot.

As Jeng and Myerson[2] note, the essential components of an effective PT tendon transfer include ensuring adequate strength of the PT tendon before transfer, harvesting maximal tendon length, performing the transfer such that the PT tendon parallels the dorsal foot, using a subcutaneous course to prevent potential tendon compression and adhesions under the extensor retinaculum, obtaining secure tendon-to-bone fixation, and ensuring appropriate rehabilitation at 6 weeks postoperatively for tendon mobilization and retraining.

A four-incision technique for PT tendon transfer for drop foot was developed by Hsu and colleagues[22,23] as a modification of Watkins original technique[13] to minimize the large anterior leg exposure. The first incision to harvest the PT tendon is made at the medial foot between the talonavicular joint and medial cuneiform. Hsu and Hoffer[22] describe the PT tendon harvest along with a periosteal flap included where the PT tendon inserts at the navicular. The PT tendon sheath is split lengthwise proximally to its retromalleolar position to facilitate transfer. A second incision at the posterior calf at the PT musculotendinous junction through its fascia is made and the distal tendon-periosteal flap is manually delivered through this incision.

With care to identify and protect the superficial peroneal nerve, a third incision is made anterior to the distal fibula to approach the interosseous membrane. A 2-cm space is created for the PT tendon transfer.[2,22,23] Care must be taken to prevent iatrogenic injury to the peroneal and posterior tibial neurovascular bundles in the deep posterior compartment. A curved Kelly clamp is then passed directly along the posterior tibia from the third (lateral) to the first (medial) incision, facilitating transfer of the PT tendon anteriorly through the window fashioned in the distal interosseous membrane. To ensure appropriate tendon gliding and minimize adhesions, it is important to make sure the actual PT muscle belly traverses the window in the interosseous membrane, and not the tendinous portion.[22]

The fourth and final incision is made over the dorsal foot at the lateral cuneiform.[2,22,23] Again, branches of the superficial peroneal nerve are protected and toe extensor tendons are mobilized and retracted. The PT tendon is then transferred from the region of the third to the fourth incision by a subcutaneous tunnel made with a long clamp from distal to proximal. After determination of appropriate tension, the distal PT tendon stump is inserted into a bone tunnel that is generally created in the lateral cuneiform, using either a suture anchor or interference screw for fixation.[2,22,23] Goh and colleagues,[24] in a cadaveric biomechanical study, determined that PT tendon transfer to the lateral cuneiform provides the most balanced, neutral ankle dorsiflexion moment.

Pinzur and colleagues[25] described and reported on their use of a combined anterior and posterior tibial tendon transfer in nine patients. The insertions of the anterior tibialis (AT) and PT tendons are transferred to a point of neutral dorsiflexion on the midfoot, which was typically the lateral cuneiform.[25] Tendo-Achilles lengthening was also performed in six of nine patients. At early follow-up (24–56 months), all nine patients were brace-free and noted subjective improvement and success of procedure.[25] Pinzur and colleagues[25] noted that, "while the surgery was initially planned to provide an active tenodesis of the ankle to resist passive ankle equinus during swing phase of gait, walking electromyography revealed 'retraining' of the transferred posterior tibial muscle to function as an active swing-phase ankle dorsiflexor muscle in seven of the nine patients."

To obviate the difficulties encountered with inadequate PT tendon length in patients with common peroneal nerve palsy, other techniques have been described.[21,26–30] Wagenaar and Louwerens,[21] using a technique described by Hansen,[26] reported on their experience with transfer of the PT tendon through the interosseous membrane with tenodesis anteriorly to the extensor tendons proximal to the ankle joint. They found good to excellent patient satisfaction in 9 of 13 feet, with no need for a previously used AFO brace in 10 of 11 feet.[21] There were three complications including one failed tendon transfer.

Postoperative protocol following PT tendon transfer generally includes a posterior splint for 2 weeks followed by a short leg walking cast, depending on other concomitant procedures performed. By 6 weeks, adequate healing has occurred to allow full mobilization and initiation of formal physical therapy for tendon retraining.[2] As Omer[20] stated, "full active dorsiflexion is rarely restored by this transfer alone; the extremity requires re-education." A night splint can be used for 3 months to prevent recurrent equinus contracture and protect the tendon transfer.

Development of an acquired flatfoot or pes planovalgus deformity has been described after PT tendon transfer.[31,32] To avoid the development of this deformity, Hansen[26] described concomitant transfer of the FDL tendon to the navicular. Equinus contracture often accompanies a drop foot deformity, necessitating either a tendo-Achilles lengthening or gastrocnemius recession to improve passive dorsiflexion.

TENDON TRANSFER PROCEDURES FOR DROP FOOT: PROXIMAL NEUROLOGIC PATHOLOGY

For patients with more proximal neurologic pathology from sciatic nerve palsy, lumbar radiculopathy, or injury to the CNS, there is often greater weakness and deformity caused by involvement of both the anterior and lateral leg compartment musculature, and sometimes even tibial nerve-innervated muscles, including the PT muscle.[2] For these types of cases, the Bridle procedure may be the best option. The Bridle procedure includes a tritendon anastomosis among the PT, AT, and peroneus longus (PL) tendons as developed by McCall and coworkers[33] for flexible equinus and equinovarus deformities. In the case of a completely flaccid foot, the Bridle procedure functions as a block to plantarflexion, and these patients may still require bracing.[3]

The PT tendon transfer portion of the Bridle procedure is performed similarly to that previously described in the prior section,[22,23] except that after transferred anteriorly through the interosseous membrane, the PT tendon is passed through a longitudinal split in the AT tendon. An additional posterolateral ankle incision (retrofibular) is made to expose the PL tendon, which is cut roughly 5 cm proximal to the distal fibula. The proximal PL stump is sewn to the peroneus brevis tendon. The distal portion of the PL tendon is pulled out from underneath the superior and inferior peroneal retinaculum and into a small incision made along the lateral hindfoot directly over the PL where it travereses the cuboid. It is then rerouted in a subcutaneous manner into the anterior-based incision and sewn to the PT and AT tendon anastomosis. All three tendons are tensioned at this level and sewn together.

McCall and coworkers[33] reported their results on 107 Bridle procedures, most performed in pediatric patients with spastic cerebral palsy. They reported 74% excellent and good results at a mean follow-up of 6.75 years.[33] The touted advantages of the original Bridle procedure over a simple PT tendon transfer include the avoidance of a tendon-to-bone attachment through a tritendon anastomosis, and a better dorsiflexion moment with the balancing effect from the AT and PL tendons.[33] There was a 12% rate of calcaneus deformity developed postoperatively, found to be caused by excessive Achilles lengthening in severely spastic patients (ie, those with diplegia and quadriplegia).[33]

Prahinski and colleagues[34] reported their results in 10 patients within the military health care system treated with Bridle transfers at a mean follow-up of 61 months. They found excellent results in low-demand patients. However, loss of dorsiflexion in high-demand patients (ie, those returning to full, active military duty) was noted and attributed to gradual stretching out of the tendon anastomosis and the loss of the tenodesis effect.[34]

Rodriguez[35,36] modified the Bridle procedure by also transferring the attachment of the PT tendon through a longitudinal slit in the AT tendon and secured to the middle cuneiform by creation of a bone tunnel. He originally reported results on 10 patients undergoing 11 Bridle procedures with a mean follow-up of 6.7 years and found all patients able to become brace-free in their ambulation with active dorsiflexion of 10° in 6 of the 10 patients.[35]

SUMMARY

The paralytic drop foot represents a challenging problem for even the most experienced orthopedic surgeon. Careful patient selection, thorough preoperative examination and planning, and application of tendon transfer biomechanical and physiologic principles outlined here can lead to successful results, either through a PT tendon transfer, Bridle transfer, or variations on these procedures. Achilles lengthening or gastrocnemius recession may also be needed at the time of tendon transfer.

REFERENCES

1. Coughlin MJ, Schon LC. Disorders of tendons. In: Coughlin MJ, Mann RA, Saltzman CL, editors. Surgery of the foot and ankle. 8th edition. Philadelphia: Mosby Elsevier, Inc; 2007. p. 1261–8.

2. Jeng C, Myerson M. The uses of tendon transfers to correct paralytic deformity of the foot and ankle. Foot Ankle Clin 2004;9:319–37.
3. Matusak SA, Baker EA, Fortin PT. The adult paralytic foot. J Am Acad Orthop Surg 2013;21:276–85.
4. Jaivin JS, Bishop JO, Braly WG, et al. Management of acquired adult dropfoot. Foot Ankle Int 1992;13:98–104.
5. Goldner JL. Surgical treatment of the paralytic foot. In: Chapman MW, editor. Operative orthopaedics, vol. 3. Philadelphia: J.B. Lippincott; 1988. p. 1799–810.
6. Mayer L. The physiological method of tendon transplantation in the treatment of paralytic drop-foot. J Bone Joint Surg Am 1937;19:389–94.
7. Bluman EM, Dowd T. The basics and science of tendon transfers. Foot Ankle Clin 2011;16:385–99.
8. Mann RA. Tendon transfers and electromyography. Clin Orthop Relat Res 1972; 85:64–6.
9. Waters RL, Frazier J, Garland DE, et al. Electromyographic gait analysis before and after operative treatment for hemiplegic equinus and equinovarus deformity. J Bone Joint Surg Am 1982;64:284–8.
10. Silver RL, de la Garza J, Rang M. The myth of muscle balance: a study of relative strengths and excursions of normal muscles about the foot and ankle. J Bone Joint Surg Br 1985;67:432–7.
11. Blix M. Die lange und die spannung des muskels. Scand Arch Physiol 1894;5: 149–206.
12. Reidy JA, Broderick TF Jr, Barr JS. Tendon transplantations in the lower extremity: a review of end results in poliomyelitis I. Tendon transplantations about the foot and ankle. J Bone Joint Surg Am 1952;34:900–8.
13. Watkins MB, Jones JB, Ryder CT Jr, et al. Transplantation of the posterior tibial tendon. J Bone Joint Surg Am 1954;36:1181–9.
14. Gunn DR, Molesworth BD. The use of tibialis posterior as a dorsiflexor. J Bone Joint Surg Am 1957;39:674–8.
15. Lipscomb PR, Sanchez JJ. Anterior transplantation of the posterior tibial tendon for persistent palsy of the common peroneal nerve. J Bone Joint Surg 1961;43: 60–6.
16. Herndon CH. Tendon transplantation at the knee and foot. Instr Course Lect 1961; 18:145–68.
17. Westin GW. Tendon transfers about the foot, ankle, and hip in the paralyzed lower extremity. J Bone Joint Surg Am 1965;47:1430–43.
18. Turner JW, Cooper RR. Anterior transfer of the tibialis posterior through the interosseous membrane. Clin Orthop Relat Res 1972;83:241–4.
19. Williams PF. Restoration of the muscle balance of the foot by transfer of the tibialis posterior. J Bone Joint Surg Br 1976;58:217–9.
20. Omer GE. Reconstructive procedures for extremities with peripheral nerve defects. Clin Orthop Relat Res 1982;(163):80–91.
21. Wagenaar FC, Louwerens JW. Posterior tibial tendon transfer: results of fixation to the dorsiflexors proximal to the ankle joint. Foot Ankle Int 2007;28:1128–42.
22. Hsu JD, Hoffer MM. Posterior tibial tendon tendon transfer anteriorly through the interosseous membrane: a modification of the technique. Clin Orthop Relat Res 1978;(131):202–4.
23. Hsu JD. Posterior tibial and anterior tibial tendon transfers for rebalancing the foot in neuromuscular disorders. Tech Foot & Ankle 2009;8:172–7.
24. Goh JC, Lee PY, Lee EH, et al. Biomechanical study on tibialis posterior tendon transfers. Clin Orthop Relat Res 1995;(319):297–302.

25. Pinzur MS, Kett N, Trilla M. Combined anteroposterior tibial tendon transfer in post-traumatic peroneal palsy. Foot Ankle Int 1988;8:271–5.
26. Hansen ST. Functional reconstruction of the foot and ankle. Philadelphia: Lippincott, Williams, and Wilkins; 2000.
27. Carayon A, Bourrell P, Bourges M, et al. Dual transfer of the posterior tibial tendon and flexor digitorum longus for drop foot. J Bone Joint Surg Am 1967;49:144–8.
28. Hove LM, Nilsen PT. Posterior tibial tendon transfer for foot-drop: 20 cases followed for 1–5 years. Acta Orthop Scand 1998;69:608–10.
29. Vigasio A, Marcoccio I, Patelli A, et al. New tendon transfer for correction of drop-foot in common peroneal nerve palsy. Clin Orthop Relat Res 2008;466:1454–66.
30. Vigasio A, Marcoccio I. Correction of drop-foot in common peroneal nerve palsy: the anterior tibialis tendon rerouting technique. Tech Foot & Ankle 2012;11:140–9.
31. Vertullo CJ, Nunley JA. Acquired flatfoot deformity following posterior tibial tendon transfer for peroneal nerve injury: a case report. J Bone Joint Surg Am 2002;84:1214–7.
32. Omid R, Thordarson DB, Charlton TP. Adult-acquired flatfoot deformity following posterior tibialis to dorsum transfer: a case report. Foot Ankle Int 2008;29:351–3.
33. McCall RE, Frederick HA, McCluskey GM, et al. The Bridle procedure: a new treatment for equinus and equinovarus deformities in children. J Pediatr Orthop 1991;11:83–9.
34. Prahinski J, McHale K, Temple T. Bridle transfer for paresis of the anterior and lateral compartment musculature. Foot Ankle Int 1996;17:615–9.
35. Rodriquez RP. The Bridle procedure in the treatment of paralysis of the foot. Foot Ankle Int 1992;13:63–9.
36. Rodriguez RP. The Bridle procedure for the treatment of dorsiflexion paralysis of the foot. Tech Foot & Ankle 2009;8:168–71.

Tendon Transfers in the Treatment of Achilles' Tendon Disorders

Steven K. Neufeld, MD[a,b], Daniel C. Farber, MD[c],*,[1]

KEYWORDS

- Tendon transfer • Achilles tendon rupture • Achilles tendinosis • V-Y advancement
- Turndown • Flexor hallucis longus tendon

KEY POINTS

- Chronic Achilles tendon disorders may benefit from tendon transfer procedures to relieve pain and improve function.
- There are numerous options to harvest in the posterior leg, including the flexor hallucis longus, flexor digitorum longus, peroneus longus and brevis, and plantaris, among others.
- The most commonly used tendon is the flexor hallucis longus, given its proximity to the Achilles, options for varying lengths, good power, and phase of action. This tendon can be harvested through the same incision as the Achilles procedure with minimal morbidity or can be harvested at the midfoot if additional tendon length is needed. Multiple studies attest to good functional results with these techniques.
- There is no available literature directly comparing different transfers, so surgeon judgment should be used in selecting the appropriate procedure. In general, good functional results and pain relief can be expected for these interventions.

PRINCIPLES OF TENDON TRANSFERS FOR ACHILLES RECONSTRUCTION

Following the principles of tendon transfers for procedures around the Achilles will help to ensure optimal outcomes.

Assessment of the soft tissue envelope is paramount. One of the most common complications of procedures around the Achilles tendon is wound-healing problems.[1] Consideration of previous incisions, infections, and scarring aids in appropriate

There are no conflicts of interest or financial interest.

[a] Orthopaedic Foot & Ankle Center of Washington, 2922 Telestar Court, Falls Church, VA 22042, USA; [b] Department of Orthopaedic Surgery, Virginia Commonwealth University, 1101 East Marshall Street, PO Box 980565 Richmond, VA 23298-0565, USA; [c] Foot and Ankle Service, Department of Orthopaedics, University of Maryland Orthopaedics and Rehabilitation Institute, University of Maryland Medical Center, University of Maryland School of Medicine, 2200 Kernan Drive, Room 1132, Baltimore, MD 21207, USA

[1] Present Address: Clinical Orthopaedic Surgery, University of Pennsylvania, Farm Journal Building, 5th Floor, 230 W. Washington Square, Philadelphia, PA 19106, USA

* Corresponding author. Clinical Orthopaedic Surgery, University of Pennsylvania, Farm Journal Building, 5th Floor, 230 W. Washington Square, Philadelphia, PA 19106

E-mail address: dcfarber@gmail.com

surgical planning, including incision location and choice of donor tendon and the potential need for staged procedures.

Although not commonly an issue for these types of Achilles' pathology, any other contractures that will affect postoperative function should be addressed with lengthening or release procedures. This may involve tendon or joint releases.

Choosing the donor tendon involves evaluation of the muscle-tendon location, strength, phase of gait, and line of pull. It is generally accepted that a transferred tendon will lose 1 grade of strength, especially if transferred out of phase. Therefore, care must be used in ensuring that the donor muscle-tendon unit has adequate preoperative power to effect the intended gain in postoperative function. In addition, the tendon transfer should not create weakness or compromise a patient's function. The relative strength compared with the native Achilles tendon of donor tendons need to be considered. For restoring Achilles tendon function, the flexor hallucis longus (FHL) and flexor digitorum longus (FDL) have the most advantageous line of pull given their location in the posterior compartment.

Biomechanical studies[2,3] have shown that the FHL tendon has relatively good strength, is an in-phase tendon, and is anatomically desirable and therefore a good donor source. The peroneal tendons are also located posterior, but in a slightly less advantageous position on the more postero-lateral aspect of the leg. The posterior tibial tendon also has a posterior muscle location, but is less commonly used because of its important native function. Furthermore, the distal muscle belly of the FHL may bring improved vascularity to the surgical area (**Table 1**).

Optimal reconstruction, regardless of the technique or specific tendon used, requires achieving normal resting tension with viable, healthy tissue.

ANATOMY
Posterior Compartment

Gastrocnemius and soleus
The gastrocnemius/soleus complex is the most dominant muscle group in the posterior leg. The gastrocnemius originates along the posterior femoral condyles, whereas the soleus arises from the proximal aspect of posterior fibula and tibia. The gastrocnemius lies posterior to the soleus, and the 2 muscles coalesce into a single tendon at 10 to 15 cm above the insertion of the Achilles into calcaneus. Branches of the S1 nerve root traveling in the tibial nerve innervate the muscles. Sural branches of

Table 1			
Relative work capacity of tendons about the ankle			
Silver et al,[3] 1985 (Based on Muscle Weights)		**Jeng et al,[2] 2012 (Based on Muscle Volume)**	
Gastroc-soleus	49	Gastroc-soleus	63.6
Post-tib	6.4	Post-tib	6.5
FHL	3.6	FHL	4.3
FDL	1.8	FDL	1.6
Peroneal Longus	2.6	Peroneal Longus	3.5

Abbreviations: FDL, flexor digitorum longus; FHL, flexor hallucis longus; Gastroc-soleus, gastrocnemius/soleus; Post-tib, posterior tibialis.
Data from Silver RL, de la Garza J, Rang M. The myth of muscle balance. A study of relative strengths and excursions of normal muscles about the foot and ankle. J Bone Joint Surg Br 1985;67(3):432–7; and Jeng CL, Thawait GK, Kwon JY, et al. Relative strengths of the calf muscles based on MRI volume measurements. Foot Ankle Int 2012;33(5):394–9.

the popliteal artery provide blood supply to the gastrocnemius, whereas the soleus receives contributions from the popliteal, posterior tibial, and sural arteries.

Plantaris

The plantaris muscle is vestigial and is seen in 97% of the population.[4] It arises from the posterior lateral intracondylar line of the femur, travels within the Achilles tendon sheath anteromedial to the Achilles, and inserts at the calcaneus just medial to the Achilles insertion. The tibial nerve also innervates it. The plantaris is rarely helpful for restoring power to the leg because of its diminutive muscle belly, but it can be helpful for providing tendon tissue to bridge a gap or reinforce a repair.

FDL

The FDL muscle originates along the posterior mid and distal tibia and inserts at the distal phalanx of the lesser toes. It is innervated by the tibial nerve (S2 nerve root) and takes its blood supply from the posterior tibial artery. The FDL is a very convenient muscle for transfer around the Achilles tendon, but lacks the power of the FHL.

FHL

The FHL is located directly anterior to the Achilles tendon. It originates from the inferior two-thirds of the posterior fibula and inserts onto the distal phalanx of the hallux. The tibial nerve provides its innervation from the S2 root. Both the peroneal and posterior tibial artery serve as its blood supply. The FHL is one of the most commonly used muscles for transfers because of its good power, phase, and proximate location to the Achilles.[5]

Posterior tibialis

This muscle arises from the superior posterior fibula and tibia and inserts onto the navicular and medial cuneiform with slips to the base of the metatarsals. It is innervated by the tibial nerve (L5 root) and receives blood supply from the sural, peroneal, and posterior tibial arteries. Although this muscle has excellent strength and is in phase with the Achilles, it is rarely used for Achilles transfer because of the morbidity of loss of its primary function as a foot invertor and supporter of the longitudinal arch of the foot.

Lateral Compartment

The peroneus longus and brevis lie in the lateral compartment along with the superficial peroneal nerve superiorly and in close proximity to the sural nerve distally. These 2 muscles are good options for transfer as they are in phase. The longus, true to its name, has potential for more length and is viewed as more expendable than the brevis tendon, especially in a cavus foot.

Peroneus longus

The longer and more powerful of these 2 muscles originates at the head of the fibula and proximal shaft and inserts on the plantar aspect of the first metatarsal base. The S1 nerve root via the common and deep peroneal nerves innervates it. The anterior tibial and peroneal arteries provide its blood supply.

In cases in which the FHL is not available, the peroneal longus tendon transfer can be a viable option. One advantage of the peroneal longus over the brevis is its relatively longer length, which can allow the transferred tendon to be doubled back on itself, adding strength to the reconstruction.[6]

Peroneus brevis

The brevis originates more inferior along the mid fibula shaft and inserts onto the base of the fifth metatarsal. It is also innervated by the S1 nerve root, but via the superficial peroneal nerve, and receives its blood supply via the peroneal artery.

Maffulli and colleagues[7] reported on the long-term follow-up of 16 patients with chronic Achilles tendon tears who were treated with an autologous peroneus brevis transfer and had good functional results.

Insertional Achilles tendinosis Although the incidence of insertional Achilles tendinopathy is not well established, it is a very common cause of posterior heel pain, especially in older, less active, less athletic, and overweight individuals. It is generally felt that the cause of Achilles tendinosis is multifactorial. At a minimum, there is a combination of decreased vascularity in the region and mechanical overload. This predisposition can then be exacerbated by poor running technique, impaired flexibility, overuse, or overload. Both hyper-pronation and cavus foot deformities have been associated with Achilles disorders.[8] The cavus foot is thought to absorb shock poorly and to place more stress on the lateral side of the Achilles tendon. In contrast, the flat foot may lead to a tight Achilles tendon and subsequent overload.

Diagnosis is based on pain, swelling, or bony enlargement at the insertion of the Achilles tendon, along with compromised function. Shoe wear can lead to mechanical discomfort, and many patients transition to backless shoes to avoid this pain. Sudden increases in activity level can also aggravate the condition. Radiographic findings often include a prominent postero-superior calcaneal tuberosity (Haglund prominence) and calcification within the Achilles insertion.[9] Mistakenly used interchangeably with tendonitis, Achilles tendinosis is characterized by fibrocartilaginous or calcifying degeneration in the area, as opposed to tendonitis, which has significant inflammation in and around the tendon. Histopathology of tendinosis demonstrates disorganization of the tendon itself with no evidence of an inflammatory reaction. Furthermore, changes in the tendon include areas of edema, hemorrhages, calcification, mucoid degeneration, and necrosis.[10–12]

The first line of treatment for insertional Achilles tendinosis should consist of conservative measures. These measures include correcting training errors, addressing malalignment, increasing flexibility, increasing muscle strength, and avoiding overuse or activities that place stress on the insertion.[12,13] Temporary immobilization in a boot walker or cast may be helpful, as is use of nonsteroidal anti-inflammatory drugs and physical therapy. Surgical treatment is considered for recalcitrant cases that have not responded to adequate conservative programs.

Established surgical treatments involve excision of the degenerative tendon, decompression of any impinging bone, and, if necessary, augmentation and reconstruction of the debrided tendon insertion. Some investigators have demonstrated good results with excision of the diseased tendon and impinging bone combined with reinsertion of the tendon by using bone anchors.[12] Many surgeons advocate transferring the FHL tendon for all surgical cases of insertional Achilles tendinosis, and others encourage the transfer in cases of extensive tendinosis greater than 50% to 75% of the tendon.[9,14] Some investigators recommend harvesting the FHL through the same posterior midline approach; however, others[15] advocate a second incision in the midfoot to gain a greater length of tendon. Tashjian and colleagues[15] showed that only 3 cm of extra length is gained if the FHL is harvested via a second incision in the midfoot at the knot of Henry. With the single posterior approach, the tibial nerve may be at risk, whereas the plantar nerves are also at risk with a midfoot incision. In the authors' experience, as well as reports by other surgeons, the single incision posterior harvest is reproducible and has excellent outcomes, faster operating room time, and little morbidity.[16–19]

There are several different surgical approaches to the insertion of the Achilles tendon. These include a central vertical Achilles splitting approach, a J-shaped incision, transverse incision (Cincinnati type), and medial and/or lateral incisions. In cases in which a tendon transfer is desired, the authors prefer a posterior vertical midline incision through the damaged Achilles tendon. This approach avoids the sural nerve and gives access to the retrocalcaneal bursa and Haglund prominence, which are excised, and the FHL tendon for transfer if necessary or desired.

Noninsertional Achilles tendinosis Noninsertional Achilles tendinosis is a common problem and presents with pain, swelling, and crepitus 3 to 5 cm above its calcaneal insertion. The occurrence is highest among runners (with poor running style) and tennis, badminton, volleyball, and soccer players. In addition, inadequate warm-up and stretching may be a contributing factor.[8,14] This is a chronic, noninflammatory degenerative process that is also seen in patients with tight gastrocnemius-soleus complex, patients with diabetes, patients who have used steroids, and in older patients.[20]

The least vascular region (vascular watershed region) is approximately 4 to 6 cm above the insertion of the Achilles into the calcaneus, which is the usual site of degeneration.[21] This area of decreased microvascularity, along with repetitive trauma, can lead to degeneration of the tendon and production of the symptoms, including pain at the area, decreased ankle range of motion, impaired gait, and decreased plantarflexion.[22]

Achilles tendinopathy presents with a thickened, often nodular area, which can be diagnosed by clinical examination. If necessary, magnetic resonance imaging (MRI) or ultrasound can be used to define the extent of tendon involvement.

Conservative treatments include rest, bracing, and avoidance of interval training, exercising up or down hills, and impact activities. Nonimpact activities, such as swimming and cycling, should be encouraged. Improving flexibility and increasing muscle strength is a primary goal. Eccentric strength exercises have been shown to improve symptoms, may reduce degenerative changes, and should be initiated early in treatment.[23]

Surgical treatment of Achilles tendinosis includes percutaneous longitudinal tenotomies,[24] gastrocnemius recession,[25,26] excision of the degenerated area and primary repair, and excision of the degenerated area with tendon augmentation of the debrided tendon segment. Removal of the entire diseased portion of the tendon is essential, as any residual degenerated tendon may increase the risk of postoperative pain. It is generally felt that if more than 50% of the Achilles tendon is involved, the FHL tendon should be transferred to augment the debrided tendon.[27] The authors typically harvest the FHL from the same posterior approach that was used for the Achilles debridement. If the gastrocnemius complex is contracted and the Silfverskiöld test is positive, it is reasonable to perform a gastrocnemius lengthening at the time of the debridement and reconstruction. The FHL muscle belly and tendon are sewn into the debrided tendon defect and secured to the calcaneus with sutures or with an interference screw through a bone tunnel.

Neglected/Chronic Achilles tendon ruptures Chronic ruptures of the Achilles tendon are a challenging problem. Patients experience pain, weakness, and loss of function when this injury is missed and the tendon does not heal or heals in an elongated position. Acute Achilles tendon ruptures can be misdiagnosed as ankle sprains when patients do not present with the classic history of a "pop" in the posterior ankle. Because other muscles, including the peroneals, plantaris, and posterior tibialis can act to plantarflex the ankle, inexperienced examiners may be fooled into believing that the Achilles is intact. However, in most cases, the Thompson test is positive and the resting position of the foot is altered when compared with the contralateral side. Ruptures not diagnosed by 4 weeks after injury may be considered chronic, as the tendon ends will have contracted in a retracted position and may no longer be reapproximated by simple manipulation.

Physical examination often reveals an atrophied calf and an inability to perform a single leg heel rise on the affected side and may be accompanied by pain in the region of the rupture site. However, manual testing may show reasonable plantarflexion strength due to use of other plantar-flexors. Patients may walk with a nonpropulsive gait on the affected side. Palpation of the area of injury may not reveal a gap, as the tendon usually fills with scar within the Achilles tendon sheath. Prone examination may show absent or diminished plantarflexion with calf squeeze and the resting position of the foot with the knee flexed is often more dorsiflexed than the contralateral side. Finally, greater maximal dorsiflexion may be present in the ruptured limb.

Conservative treatment consists of bracing with an ankle-foot orthosis. This can be a solid type or hinged with an energy-return mechanism. However, these devices can be bulky and are not always well tolerated. Physical therapy is often beneficial to maximize strength of the other plantarflexors and to learn techniques of ambulation with a weaker limb. Many patients, however, will find these results unacceptable and will desire further intervention to restore strength and decrease pain.

Surgical reconstruction is indicated to restore push-off power and the choice of the procedure relies of the amount of gap present after debridement of scar and preparation of viable tendon ends. The longer the time from initial injury, the less likely a primary end-to-end repair can be performed. Defects of 2 cm or less may be treated with primary repair; however, a small defect is rare in this setting. Defects of 2 to 8 cm are common and require advancement, turndown, and free tissue or tendon transfers to achieve continuity of the gastrocnemius-soleus complex.[28] Of these options, only a tendon transfer provides collagen material to reestablish continuity of the muscle-tendon unit as well as the potential for additional power generation for plantarflexion. The most commonly used transfer is the FHL, as it resides just anterior to the Achilles and functions in-phase with the Achilles (**Fig. 1**). It can be harvested at the posterior ankle for transfer to the calcaneus; however, more distal harvest at the midfoot will provide more tissue for reconstruction of the Achilles itself. Other tendon transfers available include the peroneals (brevis or longus) and the FDL.

Tendon Transfer Techniques for Achilles Reconstructive Procedures

FHL transfer for insertional Achilles tendonosis through a posterior approach

The patient is positioned prone on the operating table. A thigh tourniquet can be used if needed. It is helpful to have the foot positioned beyond the end of the table to allow easy dorsiflexion of the foot as needed during the procedure. Only the operative extremity need be draped. The foot is prepped to the knee. The tourniquet is insufflated after esmarch exsanguination (optional). A posterior midline incision is then performed from at least 3 cm above the insertion to the distal aspect of the insertion. More proximal incision may be necessary depending on the extent of degenerative changes in the tendon by MRI or extended later if the clinical appearance of the tendon warrants. The paratenon is preserved in the more proximal aspect of the incision. Distally, there is often degenerative tissue surrounding the Achilles and this should be excised. Dissection should be carried distal enough to visual any insertional spurs, and these can be removed with a rangeur or other instruments. The Achilles is then split longitudinally in the midline and released from its calcaneal insertion to its medial and lateral extent. In some cases, the very far lateral and far medial fibers can be left

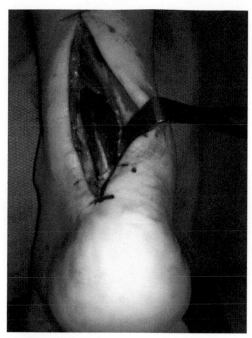

Fig. 1. The FHL muscle belly in the posterior leg.

intact, but adequate debridement should not be compromised. Full detachment does not compromise the results of the procedure, whereas inadequate debridement can be problematic. With the tendon substance visible, the diseased portion of the Achilles tendon is excised and calcified areas removed until normal tendon fibers can be visualized. The Haglund prominence is removed by using an osteotome or saw. Adequate bone should be removed to allow room for the FHL transfer and prevent any impingement. The FHL is harvested by splitting the deep fascia anterior to the Achilles. The FHL is usually easily visualized just medial to the midline at its musculo-tendinous junction (**Fig. 2**). The neurovascular bundle lies just medial to the tendon. The FHL is dissected as far distally as possible while plantarflexing the hallux. Release of the fibro-osseous tunnel along the posterior talus is necessary to gain maximum length. With the foot and hallux in maximal plantarflexion, the FHL is cut from medial to lateral to avoid neurovascular injury. The FHL tendon is secured with a suture (**Fig. 3**) and then fixed to the calcaneal insertion with the use of an interference screw,[29] bone tunnel, or suture anchors. The authors prefer interference screw fixation with tensioning via a pull-through technique. An appropriate-size tunnel is reamed through the calcaneus; however, the plantar cortex may remain intact, except the sutures from the FHL are passed through this and out the plantar heel. The FHL is maximally tensioned and the interference screw placed. The Achilles tendon is then repaired to the exposed calcaneal surface in the manner of the surgeon's preference. If desired, the healthy-appearing Achilles tendon may be anastomosed to the transferred FHL. The loss of the FHL tendon does not cause any significant postoperative morbidity to the great toe and has been shown to significantly improve function and reduce pain.[30,31] The longitudinal split in the Achilles is then repaired with #0 resorbable suture. The paratenon is closed with #3-0 resorbable suture, as is the subcutaneous tissue, followed by a nylon or monocryl skin closure.

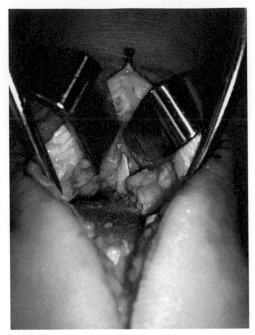

Fig. 2. The FHL visible, before harvest, through the posterior incision.

Alternative exposures include the Cincinnati incision or medial-based or lateral-based incisions. The Cincinnati incision, popularized for clubfoot releases, is a transverse incision at the level of the Achilles insertion. The medial and lateral borders of the Achilles are easily defined and the entire tendon can be released from the calcaneus to allow for tendon debridement and calcaneal exostectomy. However, harvest of the FHL is more challenging with this approach, and delayed wound healing has been noted historically; however, Maffulli and colleagues[32] reported good results with this incision for debridement alone. Medial and/or lateral incisions may also be used, but it can be difficult to access the far side for a full debridement.

FHL transfer for noninsertional Achilles tendonosis through a posterior approach
The technique for this approach is essentially the same as for insertional Achilles tendinosis, with several important differences. Most obviously, the incision will need to be

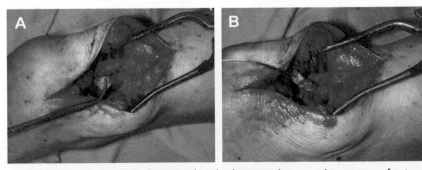

Fig. 3. (*A, B*) The FHL has been harvested and subsequently sutured to prepare for transfer.

carried more proximally to access the diseased portion of the Achilles. The authors also prefer to make this incision slightly medial to the midline in its more proximal aspect to minimize scar irritation at the posterior leg. Dissection need not be extended to the Achilles insertion, thus obviating the need for reattachment of the Achilles to the calcaneus. The paratenon is opened and the diseased Achilles tendon is identified and debrided back to healthy tissue. The FHL is harvested similar to the previous description by incising the fascia anterior to the Achilles. Once the tendon has been harvested, it may be transferred to the calcaneus through a bony tunnel and then the tendon and its muscle belly may be anastomosed to the debrided Achilles tendon. Alternatively, suture anchors, plantar button fixation, or tendon-to-tendon anastomosis may be used to secure the FHL. Routine closure, as described previously, may be used.

FHL transfer for neglected/chronic Achilles rupture with posterior harvest and V-Y advancement

The patient is positioned prone on the operating table. A thigh tourniquet may be used. It is helpful to have the foot beyond the end of the table to allow easy dorsiflexion of the foot as needed during the procedure. Only the operative extremity need be draped. The foot is prepped to the knee. The tourniquet may be insufflated or not at the surgeon's discretion. A posterior-medial incision is then performed from 4 to 5 cm proximal to the rupture to the Achilles insertion. The paratenon is then incised longitudinally and care taken to preserve this layer. In the proximal portion of the incision at the level of the musculo-tendinous junction, care must be taken to identify and protect the sural nerve that is located in the midline at this level. The rupture is then identified and the tendon released from the surrounding scar tissue. The fibrous scar is then resected as necessary to prepare viable ends. The defect between the tendon ends is assessed. Defects of less than 2 cm are rare, but may be directly approximated. Defects greater than that may benefit from a V-Y advancement or turndown procedure (**Fig. 4**).

Exposing the paratenon of the gastrocnemius and opening it to the proximal end of the musculo-tendinous junction is needed to perform the V-Y advancement. The length of the defect is measured and the "arms of the V" should be approximately twice as long as the defect itself. The "V" incision is made in the gastrocnemius fascia, leaving the underlying muscle attached to the anterior paratenon. The flap is then advanced distally by gentle stretching either using a tag suture on the end of the tendon or using a clamp (**Fig. 5**A). Slow distraction up to 5 to 10 minutes may be

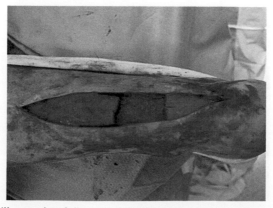

Fig. 4. Gap in Achilles tendon following debridement.

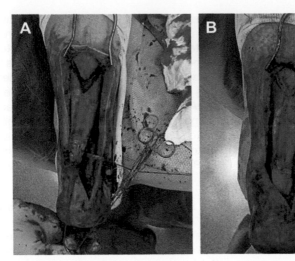

Fig. 5. (*A, B*) V-Y advancement and repair.

necessary to gain adequate length. Once the gap is closed, the repair is done using nonabsorbable braided suture. Closing the "inverted V" to a "Y" repairs the proximal portion (see **Fig. 5**B).[33] This can be done with nonabsorbable sutures. If inspection of the tendon reveals mucinous degeneration or thickening, augmentation with an FHL transfer should be considered by using either a posterior incision (as described in the technique for insertional achilles tendonosis) or midfoot harvest (as described below). A midfoot harvest in this scenario may provide additional tendon to reinforce the repair. Routine closure of the paratenon, subcutaneous layer, and skin is used.

Alternative: turndown technique
The approach is as described previously, but if there is adequate gastrocnemius fascia, longitudinal incisions are made in the fascia from 1 cm proximal to the proximal stump and extended for 2 cm longer than the measured tendon gap. This fascia is then freed from the underlying muscle and flipped distally (**Fig. 6**). Nonabsorbable sutures are placed at the apex of the turndown to prevent dissociation of the flap from the proximal stump. The turndown flap is then repaired in end-to-end fashion to the

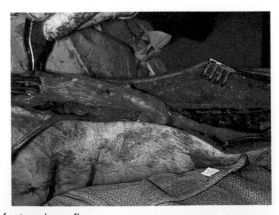

Fig. 6. Example of a turndown flap.

distal Achilles stump under desired tension. This may be further augmented with an FHL or other transfer.

Allograft or free autograft supplementation

Chronic tears of the Achilles tendon with large gaps are a surgical challenge. In addition to the FHL tendon transfer, V-Y, and turndown procedures, an allograft tendon or autograft tendon (gracillis, peroneal brevis) can be used for the reconstruction. Although the long-term results have shown continued weakness in the operative leg, patients show good functional results.[7,34]

After exposure as described previously, the tendon ends are isolated. The allograft is obtained or the autograft harvested per surgeon preference. A transverse incision is then made in the proximal stump and the allograft passed across the tendon. After ensuring adequate length of the graft on either side, the graft is secured to the tendon with nonabsorbable suture. Graft positioning is variable and depends on the length of the gap and of the graft. There should be adequate graft to loop through the proximal and distal ends and back at least once. An incision is made transversely through the distal stump and the graft placed through the tendon. The Achilles is then placed under desired tension and the loop secured both medial and lateral with nonabsorbable suture. The remaining proximal graft is then brought distal and passed in the opposite transverse direction and secured again with nonabsorbable suture. The residual graft may be cut at this point, or if adequate length remains, it can be passed proximal and fixed to the proximal tendon/muscle stump as long as that does not create excessive bulk. Closure and postoperative care are as described in the other technique descriptions.

FHL transfer midfoot harvest

If a greater length of tendon is desired for chronic ruptures or Achilles degenerative changes, the FHL can be harvested at the midfoot. The approach to the Achilles is identical to the procedures described previously. Once the FHL has been identified in the posterior incision, an incision is made along the medial foot at the glabrous skin junction. Dissection is carried above the adductor hallucis muscle and underneath the medial cuneiform. Care must be taken to cauterize or tie-off crossing veins that are almost always present to avoid a postoperative hematoma. The FHL tendon is then identified in close proximity to the flexor digitorum tendon and the medial plantar nerve. Dissection is carried as distally as needed. Protecting the adjacent neurovascular bundle, the tendon is sharply cut under visualization and pulled into the proximal wound. Fixation to the calcaneus can be made with bone anchors, interference screws, or a direct tendon through bone tunnel. The FHL tendon should be tensioned as tight as possible with the foot in plantarflexion. The authors have yet to see an overtensioned FHL transfer, as there is some creep and stretching of the transfer postoperatively. If a bone tunnel is used, a 5-mm drill hole is made at the Achilles insertion point from medial to lateral. If there is adequate length, the tendon is then woven through any remaining healthy native Achilles tendon and sutured under tension to the proximal Achilles tendon and gastrocnemius-soleus muscle. Closure is carried out per surgeon preference or as noted in the other technique descriptions.

General postoperative care A short leg splint is applied in the operating room with the foot in plantarflexion and just slight tension to the tendon transfer. The patient is encouraged to elevate the extremity as much as possible. The splint is removed approximately 7 to 14 days after surgery, sutures are removed as indicated, and a controlled ankle motion walker with Achilles lifts is applied (usually 3–4 lifts). Alternatively, the patient may be placed in a short leg cast if there are concerns about repair strength or patient compliance. Weight bearing is gradually advanced in the boot to full weight bearing at 6 weeks while sequentially removing the lifts to have the patient plantigrade by 8 weeks after surgery. Physical therapy is then instituted to regain range of motion and strength, and the patient is weaned from the boot by 10 to 12 weeks. Patients are counseled that it may take up 1 to 2 years to achieve maximal strength.

SUMMARY

Chronic Achilles tendon disorders may benefit from tendon transfer procedures to relieve pain and improve function. There are numerous options to harvest in the posterior leg, including the FHL, FDL, peroneus longus and brevis, and plantaris, among others. The most commonly used is the FHL, given its proximity to the Achilles, options for varying lengths, and good power and phase of action. This tendon can be harvested through the same incision as the Achilles procedure with minimal morbidity or can be harvested at the midfoot if additional tendon length is needed. Multiple studies attest to good functional results with these techniques.[16–19,35,36]

If the FHL is not available, then alternative tendon transfers have been described. There is no available literature directly comparing different transfers, so surgeon judgment should be used in selecting the appropriate procedure. In general, good functional results and pain relief can be expected for these interventions.

REFERENCES

1. Bruggeman NB, Turner NS, Dahm DL, et al. Wound complications after open Achilles tendon repair: an analysis of risk factors. Clin Orthop Relat Res 2004;(427):63–6.
2. Jeng CL, Thawait GK, Kwon JY, et al. Relative strengths of the calf muscles based on MRI volume measurements. Foot Ankle Int 2012;33(5):394–9.
3. Silver RL, de la Garza J, Rang M. The myth of muscle balance. A study of relative strengths and excursions of normal muscles about the foot and ankle. J Bone Joint Surg Br 1985;67(3):432–7.
4. Saxena A, Bareither D. Magnetic resonance and cadaveric findings of the incidence of plantaris tendon. Foot Ankle Int 2000;21(7):570–2.
5. Wapner KL, Pavlock GS, Hecht PJ, et al. Repair of chronic Achilles tendon rupture with flexor halluces longus tendon transfer. Foot Ankle 1993;14:443–9.
6. Char JY, Elliott AJ, Ellis SJ. Reconstruction of Achilles rerupture with peroneal longus tendon transfer. Foot Ankle Int 2013;34(6):898–903.
7. Maffulli N, Spiezia F, Pintore E, et al. Peroneus brevis tendon transfer for reconstruction of chronic tears of the Achilles tendon: a long term follow-up study. J Bone Joint Surg Am 2012;94(1):901–5.
8. Waldecker U, Hofmann G, Drewitz S. Epidemiologic investigation of 1394 feet: coincidence of hindfoot malalignment and Achilles tendon disorders. Foot Ankle Surg 2012;18(2):119–23.
9. DeOrio MJ, Easley ME. Surgical strategies: insertional Achilles tendinopathy. Foot Ankle Int 2008;29(5):542–50.
10. Clement DB, Taunton JE, Smart GW. Achilles tendinitis and peritendinitis: etiology and treatment. Am J Sports Med 1984;12:179–84.
11. Sorosky B, Press J, Piastaras C, et al. The practical management of Achilles tendinopathy. Clin J Sport Med 2004;14:40–4.
12. Maffulli N, Testa V, Capasso G, et al. Calcific insertional Achilles tendinopathy. Replacement with bone anchors. Am J Sports Med 2004;32:174–82.

13. Astrom M, Gentz CF, Nilsson P, et al. Imaging in chronic Achilles tendinopathy: a comparison of ultrasonography, magnetic resonance imaging and surgical findings in 27 histologically verified cases. Skeletal Radiol 1996;25:615–20.
14. Hartog BD. Insertional Achilles tendinosis: pathogenesis and treatment. Foot Ankle Clin 2009;14:639–50.
15. Tashjian RZ, Hur J, Sullivan RJ, et al. Flexor hallucis longus transfer for repair of chronic Achilles tendinopathy. Foot Ankle Int 2003;24(9):673–6.
16. Will RE, Galey SM. Outcome of single incision flexor hallucis longus transfer for chronic Achilles tendinopathy. Foot Ankle Int 2009;30(4):315–7.
17. Elias I, Raikin SM, Besser MP, et al. Outcomes of chronic insertional Achilles tendinosis using FHL autograft through single incision. Foot Ankle Int 2009;30(3): 197–204.
18. Hahn F, Meyer P, Maiwald C, et al. Treatment of chronic Achilles tendinopathy and ruptures with flexor hallucis tendon transfer: clinical outcome and MRI findings. Foot Ankle Int 2008;29(8):794–802.
19. Martin RL, Manning CM, Carcia CR, et al. An outcome study of chronic Achilles tendinosis after excision of the Achilles tendon and flexor hallucis longus tendon transfer. Foot Ankle Int 2005;26(9):691–7.
20. Holmes GB, Lin J. Etiologic factors associated with symptomatic Achilles tendinopathy. Foot Ankle Int 2006;27:952–9.
21. Chen TM, Rozen WM, Pan WR, et al. The arterial anatomy of the Achilles tendon: anatomical study and clinical implications. Clin Anat 2009;22(3):377–85.
22. Jones DC. Tendon disorders of the foot and ankle. J Am Acad Orthop Surg 1993; 1(2):87–94.
23. Silbernagel KG, Thomeé R, Thomeé P, et al. Eccentric overload training for patients with chronic Achilles tendon pain—a randomized controlled study with reliability testing of the evaluation methods. Scand J Med Sci Sports 2001; 11(4):197–206.
24. Maffulli N, Testa V, Capasso G, et al. Results of percutaneous longitudinal tenotomy for Achilles tendinopathy in middle- and long-distance runners. Am J Sports Med 1997;25:835–40.
25. Gurdezi S, Kohls-Gatzoulis J, Solan MC. Results of proximal medial gastrocnemius release for Achilles tendinopathy. Foot Ankle Int 2013;34(10):1364–9.
26. Kiewiet NJ, Holthusen SM, Bohay DR, et al. Gastrocnemius recession for chronic noninsertional Achilles tendinopathy. Foot Ankle Int 2013;34(4):481–5.
27. Den Hartog BD. Flexor hallucis longus transfer for chronic Achilles tendinosis. Foot Ankle Int 2003;24:233–7.
28. Villarreal AD, Andersen CR, Panchbhavi VK. A survey on management of chronic Achilles tendon ruptures. Am J Orthop (Belle Mead NJ) 2012;41(3):126–31.
29. Cottom JM, Hyer CF, Berlet GC, et al. Flexor hallucis tendon transfer with an interference screw for chronic Achilles tendinosis: a report of 62 cases. Foot Ankle Spec 2008;1(5):280–7.
30. Coul R, Flavin R, Stephens MM. Flexor hallucis longus tendon transfer: evaluation of postoperative morbidity. Foot Ankle Int 2003;12:931–4.
31. Schon LC, Shores JL, Faro FD, et al. Flexor hallucis longus tendon transfer in treatment of Achilles tendinosis. J Bone Joint Surg Am 2013;95(1):54–60.
32. Maffulli N, Del Buono A, Testa V, et al. Safety and outcome of surgical debridement of insertional Achilles tendinopathy using a transverse (Cincinnati) incision. J Bone Joint Surg Br 2011;93(11):1503–7.
33. Abraham E, Pankovich AM. Neglected rupture of the Achilles tendon: treatment by V-Y tendinous flap. J Bone Joint Surg Am 1975;57:253–5.

34. Maffulli N, Spiezia F, Testa V, et al. Free gracilis tendon graft for reconstruction of chronic tears of the Achilles tendon. J Bone Joint Surg Am 2012;94(10):906–10.
35. Rahm S, Spross C, Gerber F, et al. Operative treatment of chronic irreparable Achilles tendon ruptures with large flexor hallucis longus tendon transfers. Foot Ankle Int 2013;34(8):1100–10.
36. Yeoman TF, Brown MJ, Pillai A. Early post-operative results of neglected tendo-Achilles rupture reconstruction using short flexor hallucis longus tendon transfer: a prospective review. Foot (Edinb) 2012;22(3):219–23.

Salvage Options for Peroneal Tendon Ruptures

Emmanouil D. Stamatis, MD, FHCOS, PhD*,
Georgios C. Karaoglanis, MD

KEYWORDS

- Peroneal tendons • Ruptures • Tears • Salvage • Tendon transfer • Allograft

KEY POINTS

- Irreparable peroneal tendon ruptures or completely unsalvageable tendons after failure of previously attempted repairs are encountered rarely.
- The choice of treatment strategy depends on the presence of a functioning tendon or tendons and the viability and excursion of the peroneal musculature.
- When one irreparable tendon is encountered the salvage options include either tenodesis or bridging of the defect using allografts or autografts.
- When both tendons are irreparable the salvage options include FDL or FHL tendon transfer.
- All treatment strategies should be augmented, depending on the underlying pathophysiology, by peroneal tendon stabilization, lateral ligament repair, and/or hindfoot correction procedures.

INTRODUCTION

Peroneal tendon pathology including fraying, longitudinal fissuring, partial and full-thickness tears, or even complete rupture has been identified as a major cause of persistent posterolateral or lateral hindfoot pain, and substantial functional disability.[1–3]

The incidence of peroneal tendon tears in the general population is unknown, because the only available figures come from two cadaveric studies by Sobel and colleagues,[4,5] who reported the striking different incidences of 11.3% and 37% in elderly patients. The exact incidence is somewhere between the high numbers of the cadaveric studies and the very small numbers reported clinically in the spare retrospective series.

No benefits in any form have been received or will be received from a commercial party related directly or indirectly to the subject of this article. The views expressed in this article are those of the authors and do not reflect the official policy or position of the Department of Defence of the Hellenic Government.
Orthopaedic Department, 401 General Army Hospital, Thrakis 23 Street, Athens 17121, Greece
* Corresponding author.
E-mail address: mstamatis66@yahoo.com

Foot Ankle Clin N Am 19 (2014) 87–95
http://dx.doi.org/10.1016/j.fcl.2013.10.006
1083-7515/14/$ – see front matter © 2014 Elsevier Inc. All rights reserved.

foot.theclinics.com

Although since the late 1980s and early 1990s there was an increased awareness of the pathophysiology and diagnosis of peroneal tendon tears and focused attention in the literature regarding treatment options,[6–12] it was not until 1998 when Krause and Brodsky[13] first proposed operative treatment criteria based on the severity of tendon involvement.

Since their recommendation, several reports with favorable outcomes have been published when surgical treatment is used. Unfortunately, all studies reporting on the surgical management of peroneal tendon tears are either small retrospective reviews[14–18] (level of evidence IV) or case reports[19–21] (level of evidence V); thus, there is insufficient evidence to recommend for or against any specific treatment strategy.

Irreparable peroneal tendon tears or completely unsalvageable tendons after failure of previously attempted repairs are rare, and thus there is a striking lack of high-level evidence to guide the management of these complex injuries (**Table 1**).

The apparent rarity of these pathologic entities along with the lack of adequate evidence because of nonuniformity of proposed treatment options creates a challenging therapeutic problem. A critical review of the available literature[22–27] could be of significant educational value for the foot and ankle surgeon confronting similar cases, enabling him or her to accurately diagnose and assess the injury pattern and choose the type of surgical strategy and rehabilitation regimen to enhance a good functional outcome.

Table 1
Articles reporting data on salvage of peroneal tendon ruptures

Article	No. of Patients	No. of Patients with One Irreparable Tendon	No. of Patients with Two Irreparable Tendons	Type of Procedure (No. of Patients)
Wapner et al,[27] 2006	7	N/A	7	Staged FHL transfer (7)
Redfern & Myerson,[26] 2004	28	1	12	Staged FDL transfer (1) One-stage FDL transfer (3) Tenodesis (1) Staged allograft (3) One-stage allograft (1) Peroneus longus transfer to distal stump of peroneus brevis or fifth metatarsal (4)
Jockel & Brodsky,[23] 2013	8	N/A	8	One-stage FHL transfer (4) One-stage FDL transfer (4)
Rapley et al,[25] 2010	11	11	N/A	Repair with "gap jump" acellular dermal matrix allograft (11)
Mook et al,[24] 2013	14	10	4	One-stage tendon allograft reconstruction One tendon only (13 patients) Two tendons (1)
Krause & Brodsky,[13] 1998	20	9	N/A	Tenodesis (9)

The possible scenarios of peroneal tendon tears that could be encountered in the clinical setting include (1) only one peroneal tendon is involved and it is amenable to repair; (2) both tendons are compromised but they are functional after repair; (3) one peroneal tendon is severely compromised and unsalvageable, whereas the other is either intact or repairable; or (4) both tendons are unsalvageable. This article discusses the proposed treatment strategies for reconstruction of the unsalvageable tendons along with any concomitant procedures dealing with associated pathology (deficient collateral ligaments, peroneal retinaculum, peroneal sulcus, and varus hindfoot) predisposing to tendon impairment.

SALVAGE OPTIONS FOR ONE IRREPARABLE PERONEAL TENDON

Despite the rarity of peroneal tendon tears, repair or tendon debridement and tubularization had been proposed as the preferred treatment option.[6–12] The issue arising from these early reports was that there were no definite guidelines of what is considered adequate and viable tendon remnant amenable to repair.

Krause and Brodsky[13] first proposed a classification system to guide treatment decision-making. Their simple system was based on the transverse width (cross-sectional area) of viable tendon remaining after debridement of the involved portion, presuming that the remaining tendon is free of degeneration and longitudinal tears. Thus, if 50% or more of the cross-sectional area of the tendon was viable after debridement (Grade I) then these lesions could be treated with tendon repair. In contrast, if less than 50% of the tendon was viable after debridement (Grade II) then these lesions should be treated with segmental resection of the heavily involved tendon and tenodesis.

Although the authors[13] proposed a reasonable treatment option for the irreparable tears of one peroneal tendon, other authors elected to treat this difficult problem by trying to preserve the functional integrity of muscle-tendon unit, which is obviously sacrificed with a tenodesis, by spanning the defect after impaired tendon resection with tendon allograft[24] or acellular dermal matrix allograft.[25]

Salvage of Peroneal Tendon Rupture with Tenodesis

Tenodesis of a severely compromised peroneal tendon to the adjacent usable one or even to the cuboid or the calcaneus had been anecdotally reported as a salvage procedure for peroneus longus ruptures[3,12] and in two patients with a peroneus brevis tear.[14]

Krause and Brodsky[13] were the first to report on the outcome of a small series of nine patients who underwent such a salvage procedure for an irreparable peroneus brevis tear comparing their outcome with that of a second small group of 11 patients who underwent debridement and repair. Despite the fact that the study was retrospective and that the available numbers were small, not allowing for powerful statistical analysis, the authors concluded that the subjective and objective results were not substantially different between the two groups.

They proposed proximal and distal tenodeses of the peroneus brevis to longus, cautioning for placement of the proximal and distal sites, 3 to 4 cm above and 5 to 6 cm below the tip of the lateral malleolus, respectively, to avoid fibular impingement. They also stressed that such an approach should be augmented by correcting the underlying pathologies predisposing to tendon impairment, which according to their opinion were mainly chronic subluxation of the tendons and/or deficient peroneal groove.

Although in the latter study the authors did not encounter concomitant hindfoot malalignment or ankle instability, this is not always the case when dealing with severely compromised peroneal tendons. Redfern and Myerson[26] and Steel and DeOrio[18] reported that in the presence of varus hindfoot or lateral ligament deficiency of the ankle joint, they combined the tenodesis with a lateralizing calcaneal osteotomy or a lateral ligament reconstruction procedure, respectively, to eliminate anatomic factors that may contribute to peroneal tendons pathology.

Salvage of Peroneal Tendon Rupture with Allograft Reconstruction

Although tenodesis is a relatively simple and less technically demanding procedure with relatively good functional results, there are still issues arising from such an approach. Almost 50% of the patients did not resume full activities, whereas almost two-thirds reported activity-related pain.[13]

To preserve the muscle-tendon unit in continuity enhancing the maximum function, Mook and colleagues[24] proposed the bridging of an intercalary segment tendon defect using tendon allografts. In their small retrospective series of 14 patients,[14] seven presented with extended nonsalvageable pathology of the peroneus brevis only. The other seven patients presented with impairment of both tendons, but after debridement and intraoperative assessment the authors encountered one irreparable tendon in four, and both tendons severely impaired and unusable in three. The 11 patients with one irreparable tendon were treated with the use of either peroneal or semitendinosus tendon allografts. In all cases the allograft was secured to the distal native tendon stump with a Pulvertaft weave or in the rare instance of inadequate distal stump, to the fifth metatarsal using 3.5-mm suture anchors. After setting the appropriate muscle-tendon unit tension a Pulvertaft weave was also used to secure the proximal part of the allograft to the remaining healthy proximal stump.

The authors also stressed the importance of intraoperative assessment of adequate proximal stump excursion as an indicator that the muscle is still functional and has not become contracted. It is also notable that more than 50% of the patients in their series underwent concomitant surgical procedures to address coexisting pathology (deficient peroneal groove, lateral ligament deficiency, and varus hindfoot) predisposing to peroneal tendon impairment.

The mean follow-up was relatively short (17 months), and the authors reported that all patients returned to their preinjury activity levels, and their functional scores improved significantly.

The main issues associated with the use of allografts are the risk of infectious disease transmission (minimal), the high cost, the risks of inferior mechanical properties, and the prolonged incorporation time caused by the sterilization process. Previous studies have documented the decline in durability and function of allograft tendons in other anatomic locations.[28]

The authors, however, relying on their anecdotal experience, reported that they have not observed any adverse effects related to the use of allografts by means of reduced biomechanical properties. They attributed their observation to the sterilization formula that had been used to disinfect all the allografts used in their study.[24] However, these observations have not been documented with evidence.

In their opinion, the use of autograft tendons is an alternative that could potentially reduce the cost and outweigh the potential biologic disadvantages of allografts, and it should be discussed with the patient taking into account all the parameters.[24]

Salvage of Peroneal Tendon Rupture with Acellular Dermal Matrix Allograft

The use of acellular dermal matrix allografts for the repair of severely compromised tendons or ruptures with segmental defects has been reported as an alternative in the shoulder demonstrating good initial clinical results.

Rapley and colleagues[25] reported use of this novel treatment modality to augment repairs of severely compromised tendons or to bridge segmental defects. Their small retrospective series of 11 patients included four patients with previous tenodesis, four patients with segmental tendon loss, and three patients with involvement of more than 50% of the tendon. All four previous tenodeses were taken down and each tendon was isolated and, similar to the four patients with segmental defect, the gap was bridged with a properly tubularized acellular dermal matrix allograft, wrapped around the defect and secured with sutures proximally and distally. The three patients with extended pathology (more than 50%) were treated with suturing of the tendon remnants and augmentation of the repair with tubularized acellular dermal matrix allograft, which was wrapped around. All the patients underwent concomitant surgery by means of fibular sulcus deepening.

The follow-up was rather short (17 months) and the authors reported impressive clinical results. The potential advantages supporting their approach are the preservation of a functional muscle-tendon unit, even taking down a previous tenodesis, and the avoidance of use of tendon allografts with their potential side effects or autografts thus reducing the morbidity to the donor site. However, the issue arising from their study is the excellent clinical outcome obtained with the use of a foreign material to bridge gaps of the peroneal tendons, which are notorious for their low potential for healing because of poor vascularity.

SALVAGE OPTIONS FOR BOTH IRREPARABLE PERONEAL TENDONS

Ruptures of both the peroneal tendons have rarely been documented, and studies reporting on the treatment options are limited to a few case reports[6,16,20–22] or very small retrospective series.[23,24,26,27] Irreparable tears of both tendons are encountered even more rarely,[22,23,26,27] and as a consequence there are sparse treatment guidelines for these complex pathologies (see **Table 1**). Nonusable or irreparable peroneal tendon tears can also be encountered in clinical practice, in a small subset of patients who had previous surgical procedures that did not work.[27]

Redfern and Myerson[26] proposed, through a rather heterogeneous case series, a very useful treatment algorithm (**Fig. 1**) for peroneal tendon surgery based on the intraoperative assessment of the extent of tendon pathology. Thus, type I tears include those where both tendons are usable, type II tears include those where one of the tendons is repairable or usable, and type III tears include those where both tendons are irreparable. They further subclassified that latter type into IIIa and IIB, depending on the absence or presence of proximal muscle excursion, respectively. Their recommendation was that type IIIa ruptures should be treated with a tendon transfer, because there was no available muscle belly to be used. However, type IIIb ruptures were considered amenable to reconstruction with tendon allograft in one stage or as staged procedures depending on the absence or presence of scar tissue.

Salvage of Both Peroneal Tendon Ruptures with Allografts

Redfern and Myerson,[26] in the presence of two irreparable tendons, performed isolated reconstruction of the peroneus brevis as a staged procedure in three patients, and as a single procedure in one patient. In all staged procedures, and during the first surgery, they intraoperatively confirmed that there was residual proximal muscle excursion and through two small incisions inserted a Hunter rod to enhance formation of a tendon pseudosheath. During the second stage a hamstring allograft was inserted with the aim of the silicone rod. All four patients demonstrated significant improvement of their functional scores, but the authors surprisingly noted that the staged

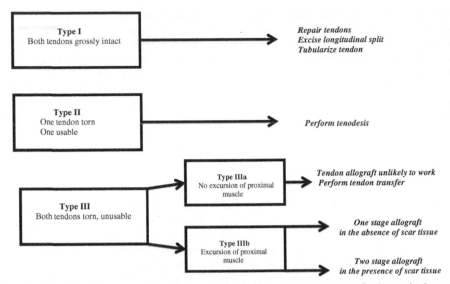

Fig. 1. Algorithm for peroneal tendon surgery based on intraoperative findings. (*Adapted from* Redfern D, Myerson M. The management of concomitant tears of the peroneus longus and brevis tendons. Foot Ankle Int 2004;25(10):699; with permission.)

procedures produced substantially more scarring than expected. Based on that observation they were biased toward extending the indications for one-stage procedures. Finally, they stressed the importance of treating at the time of tendon repair any associated pathology contributing to tendon tears.

Mook and colleagues[24] also reported on the use of tendon allografts in three patients where they encountered extended pathology to both tendons. In one patient they reconstructed both tendons, whereas in the other two they reconstructed either the peroneus brevis or the peroneus longus. They pointed out that reconstruction of peroneus longus should only be performed in cases where the tear was proximal enough to allow for an adequate Pulvertaft weave, without the need for further dissection on the plantar aspect of the foot, which would potentially increase the morbidity.

It is apparent that the use of tendon allografts, although commonly proposed, is not supported by adequate data. The few cases reported in the previously mentioned small series, despite the reported good outcomes, do not lend themselves to the proposal of this treatment modality with acceptable level of recommendation.

Salvage of Both Peroneal Tendon Ruptures with Tendon Transfer

Borton and colleagues[22] initially described the flexor digitorum longus (FDL) tendon transfer as a reconstruction method of concomitant irreparable peroneal tendon tears. Redfern and Myerson[26] subsequently reported on the use of FDL tendon transfer for the treatment of four patients with type IIIa concomitant ruptures, as they were described in their proposed algorithm. Wapner and colleagues[27] reported on the staged reconstruction of seven patients with chronic ruptures of both peroneal tendons, caused by failed previous surgeries, using the flexor hallucis longus (FHL) tendon transfer in a staged fashion. Finally, Jockel and Brodsky[23] reported on the single-stage FDL or FHL transfer for the treatment of similar pathology in eight patients. All tendons were similarly harvested at the level of knot of Henry to ensure adequate length. Through a second small incision made posteromedially just above the ankle joint, the tendon was retrieved and mobilized while ensuring that the neurovascular bundle was adequately protected. In all cases the tendon was then passed from medial to lateral around the posterior aspect of the tibia and fibula, and subsequently attached either to the base of the fifth metatarsal[23] by a drill hole, or to the distal stump of the peroneus brevis using a Pulvertaft weave.[26,27]

The reported functional results from all authors are rather encouraging, but a careful approach of the reports may generate several issues, discussed next.

Which patients are the appropriate candidates for a tendon transfer?

According to Sammarco,[2] Redfern and Myerson,[26] and Wapner and colleagues,[27] a tendon transfer should be used *only* in cases where both tendons present with extensive pathology constituting them irreparable, and there is also no proximal muscle excursion. Jockel and Brodsky[23] did not agree with the latter approach, and they clearly stated that it is very challenging to reliably assess the proximal muscle excursion in the anesthetized patient and to reproduce this kind of examination. Practically, they rejected the differentiation between types IIIa and IIIb, thus proposing tendon transfer for all patients with concomitant, severe peroneal ruptures. To further support their proposal for routine use of a tendon transfer against the possible use of allografts as a treatment alternative, they highlighted previous studies that have documented the decline in durability and function of allograft tendons in other locations.[28]

Which is the most appropriate tendon to be transferred, the FHL or the FDL?

Theoretically, either transfer is reasonable because both tendons are in-phase donors. The only study where there is a direct clinical comparison, even with very few reported cases, is that by Jockel and Brodsky[23] who reported good outcomes with both tendons. However, the authors favor FHL transfer because the patients who had undergone the later transfer demonstrated improved eversion strength, higher mean American Orthopaedic Foot and Ankle Society postoperative scores, and better subjective assessment of their functional status. Further, Silver and colleagues[29] using cadaver dissections calculated the strength and work percentage of the FHL to be twice that of the FDL, with both tendons having similar excursion potential. Jeng and colleagues[30] determined the relative work capacity of calf musculature in vivo using magnetic resonance imaging measurements and concluded that the FHL was the appropriate tendon for peroneal reconstruction.

What is the appropriate timing for a tendon transfer?

Jockel and Brodsky[23] and Redfern and Myerson[26] preferred one-stage procedures, whereas Wapner and colleagues[27] proposed a staged reconstruction. The reader should keep in mind the interesting observations that were reported by the authors. Redfern and Myerson[26] reported that even with minimal incisions and atraumatic technique they encountered excessive scar tissue formation during the second stage, favoring the one-stage procedure. Additionally, Jockel and Brodsky[23] reported that the presence of excessive scarring and loss of adequate tendon sheath caused by previous surgeries or chronicity of the pathology is a scenario that they never encountered intraoperatively; thus, one-stage surgery was strongly recommended. The reader should also keep in mind that the reconstructions reported by Wapner and colleagues[27] were performed in a special subset of patients with multiple previous surgeries with subsequent extended fibrosis and complete absence of peroneal sheath. The advantage of the use of a silicone Hunter rod as a staged procedure in revision cases is the re-creation of a viable tendon pseudosheath producing a fluid resembling synovial fluid, thus enhancing the gliding motion of the transferred tendon.

Is there a need for concomitant procedures?
FHL or FDL tendon transfers are able to restore the function of only the peroneus brevis. Theoretically the absence of peroneus longus function results in net inversion of the hindfoot by the posterior tibial tendon. In chronic cases, because the peroneus longus is more than twice as strong as the peroneus brevis, this imbalance may lead to varus hindfoot. Wapner and colleagues[27] reported that at follow-up they did not notice any measurable morbidity from the latter muscle imbalance, stating that there was not a reasonable explanation for that observation, despite the fact that they had performed the FHL transfer as an isolated procedure. Jockel and Brodsky[23] and Redfern and Myerson[26] combined their transfers with concomitant procedures, namely calcaneal osteotomy for hindfoot realignment, lateral ankle ligament reconstruction, or dorsiflexion osteotomy of the first metatarsal, either to correct any existing deformity or to create a favorable mechanical environment for the transfer.

SUMMARY

Irreparable peroneal tendon tears or completely unsalvageable tendons after failure of previously attempted repairs are rare; thus, there is insufficient evidence to recommend for or against any specific treatment strategy. The clinical scenarios necessitating salvage reconstructive procedures are either of one severely compromised and unsalvageable peroneal tendon, whereas the other is either intact/repairable, or of both unsalvageable tendons. In the setting of one irreparable tendon, salvage options include tenodesis, or spanning of the defect with tendon allograft or acellular dermal matrix allograft. Tenodesis is an easy and reproducible procedure, but the use of allografts is theoretically more advantageous, because it preserves the functional integrity of the muscle-tendon unit. The use of allografts includes the risks of infectious disease transmission, inferior mechanical properties, and the prolonged incorporation time reducing their durability and function. One-stage FHL tendon transfer seems to represent a reasonable salvage procedure in cases where both peroneal tendons are unusable.

REFERENCES

1. Sammarco GJ, DiRaimondo CV. Chronic peroneus brevis tendon tears. Foot Ankle 1989;9(4):163–70.
2. Sammarco GJ. Peroneal tendon injuries. Orthop Clin North Am 1994;25(1): 135–45.
3. Sammarco GJ. Peroneus longus tears: acute and chronic. Foot Ankle Int 1995; 16(5):245–53.
4. Sobel M, Bohne WH, Levy ME. Longitudinal attrition of the peroneus brevis tendon in the fibular groove: an anatomic study. Foot Ankle 1990;11(3):124–8.
5. Sobel M, DiCarlo EF, Bohne WH, et al. Longitudinal splitting of the peroneus brevis tendon: an anatomic and histologic study of cadaver material. Foot Ankle 1991;12(3):165–70.
6. Bassett FH 3rd, Speer KP. Longitudinal rupture of the peroneal tendons. Am J Sports Med 1993;21(3):354–7.
7. Khoury NJ, el-Khoury GY, Saltzman CL, et al. Peroneus longus and brevis tendon tears: MR imaging evaluation. Radiology 1996;200(3):833–41.
8. Larsen E. Longitudinal rupture of the peroneus brevis tendon. J Bone Joint Surg Br 1987;69(2):340–1.
9. Munk RL, Davis PH. Longitudinal rupture of the peroneus brevis tendon. J Trauma 1976;16(10):803–6.

10. Saxena A, Pham B. Longitudinal peroneal tendon tears. J Foot Ankle Surg 1997; 36(3):173–9.
11. Shoda E, Kurosaka M, Yoshiya S, et al. Longitudinal ruptures of the peroneal tendons. A report of a rugby player. Acta Orthop Scand 1991;62(5):491–2.
12. Thompson FM, Patterson AH. Rupture of the peroneus longus tendon. J Bone Joint Surg Am 1989;71(2):293–5.
13. Krause JO, Brodsky JW. Peroneus brevis tendon tears: pathophysiology, surgical reconstruction, and clinical results. Foot Ankle Int 1998;19(5):271–9.
14. Dombek MF, Lamm BM, Saltrick K, et al. Peroneal tendon tears: a retrospective review. J Foot Ankle Surg 2003;42(5):250–8.
15. Grant TH, Kelikian AS, Jereb SE, et al. Ultrasound diagnosis of peroneal tendon tears. A surgical correlation. J Bone Joint Surg Am 2005;87(8):1788–94.
16. Pelet S, Saglini M, Garofalo R, et al. Traumatic rupture of both peroneal longus and brevis tendons. Foot Ankle Int 2003;24(9):721–3.
17. Saxena A, Cassidy A. Peroneal tendon injuries: an evaluation of 49 tears in 41 patients. J Foot Ankle Surg 2003;42(4):215–20.
18. Steel MW, DeOrio JK. Peroneal tendon tears: return to sports after operative treatment. Foot Ankle Int 2007;28(1):49–54.
19. Cooper ME, Selesnick FH, Murphy BJ. Partial peroneus longus tendon rupture in professional basketball players: a report of 2 cases. Am J Orthop 2002;31(12): 691–4.
20. Verheyen CP, Bras J, van Dijk CN. Rupture of both peroneal tendons in a professional athlete. A case report. Am J Sports Med 2000;28(6):897–900.
21. Wind WM, Rohrbacher BJ. Peroneus longus and brevis rupture in a collegiate athlete. Foot Ankle Int 2001;22(2):140–3.
22. Borton DC, Lucas P, Jomha NM, et al. Operative reconstruction after transverse rupture of the tendons of both peroneus longus and brevis. Surgical reconstruction by transfer of the flexor digitorum longus tendon. J Bone Joint Surg Br 1998; 80(5):781–4.
23. Jockel JR, Brodsky JW. Single-stage flexor tendon transfer for the treatment of severe concomitant peroneus longus and brevis tendon tears. Foot Ankle Int 2013;34(5):666–72.
24. Mook WR, Parekh SG, Nunley JA. Allograft reconstruction of peroneal tendons: operative technique and clinical outcomes. Foot Ankle Int 2013;34(9):1212–20.
25. Rapley JH, Crates J, Barber A. Mid-substance peroneal tendon defects augmented with an acellular dermal matrix allograft. Foot Ankle Int 2010;31(2): 136–40.
26. Redfern D, Myerson M. The management of concomitant tears of the peroneus longus and brevis tendons. Foot Ankle Int 2004;25(10):695–707.
27. Wapner KL, Taras JS, Lin SS, et al. Staged reconstruction for chronic rupture of both peroneal tendons using Hunter rod and flexor hallucis longus tendon transfer: a long-term followup study. Foot Ankle Int 2006;27(8):591–7.
28. Leopold SS, Greidanus N, Paprosky WG, et al. High rate of failure of allograft reconstruction of the extensor mechanism after total knee arthroplasty. J Bone Joint Surg Am 1999;81(11):1574–9.
29. Silver RL, de la Garza J, Rang M. The myth of muscle balance: a study of relative strengths and excursions of normal muscles about the foot and ankle. J Bone Joint Surg Br 1985;67(3):432–7.
30. Jeng CL, Thawait GK, Kwon JY, et al. Relative strengths of the calf muscles based on MRI volume measurements. Foot Ankle Int 2012;33(5):394–9.

Spastic Foot and Ankle Deformities: Evaluation and Treatment

Brandon W. King, MD, David J. Ruta, MD, Todd A. Irwin, MD*

KEYWORDS

- Spastic foot and ankle deformities • SPLATT • Equinovarus

KEY POINTS

- Spastic equinovarus is the most common foot and ankle deformity following cerebral vascular accidents.
- Dynamic electromyogram is the most important preoperative tool in planning surgical correction.
- Surgery should be considered when the patient is at a plateau of neurologic improvement with goals of producing a balanced, functional foot, minimize brace wear, pain relief, callus/ulcer prevention, facilitating hygiene, and/or positioning in a wheelchair.
- Operative intervention has been shown to improve ambulatory status and decrease necessity of brace wear.

INTRODUCTION

Traumatic brain injuries (TBIs) and strokes, or cerebral vascular accidents (CVAs), can have profound effects on both the individual and society as a whole. The most recent American Heart Association statistics report the annual adult incidence of CVAs in the United States to be nearly 800,000, of which more than half survive,[1-3] thereby making it the leading cause of serious long-term disability in the United States.[1,4] TBIs are even more common, with an incidence of 1.5 million per year.[5] In addition to frequent cognitive deficits, residual musculoskeletal disabilities are common, with 30% unable to ambulate without assistance.[1] TBIs and CVAs are therefore the leading causes of adult spastic foot and ankle deformities.[4,6] Similar deformities are also common in cerebral palsy with similar treatment strategies, although most are addressed in childhood.

Disclosures: None (B.W. King and D.J. Ruta); I and/or my spouse/significant partner/immediate family member have the following financial relationships: Smith and Nephew – consultant, advisor; Saunders/Mosby-Elsevier – financial support from publisher (T.A. Irwin).
Department of Orthopaedic Surgery, University of Michigan Hospital System, 2912 Taubman Center, Ann Arbor, MI 48109, USA
* Corresponding author.
E-mail address: tirwin@med.umich.edu

CAUSE

Spastic foot deformities are caused by selectively increased muscle tone that disturbs the physiologic agonist-antagonist balance of the lower extremity musculature. Head or spinal cord trauma, ischemia, hemorrhage, demyelinating disease, infection, and inflammatory diseases are all potential causes.[4,6,7] Spasticity stems from an upper motor neuron disruption along the descending corticospinal tract, with variability in both specific location and cause.[4,8] For instance, a CVA in the distribution of the anterior cerebral artery results in hemiparesis or hemiplegia, and there is even greater severity with brainstem involvement.[4,6] The result is a loss of the normal inhibitory signal from interneurons, producing hyperexcitability of motor neurons. Exaggeration of the muscle-tendon stretch reflex occurs, causing a velocity-dependent increase in muscular tone.[4] In the lower extremity, the extensors are typically more affected, in contrast to greater flexor involvement in the upper extremity.[4] The spasticity can also be affected by temperature and emotion.[4,9]

Cerebral palsy is a static encephalopathy secondary to a nonprogressive insult to the developing brain. The resultant musculoskeletal deformities, however, are progressive, in that the growth of bones outpaces that of associated tendons.[4] With increasing age and growth, the tendons are no longer able to compensate, and permanent structural deformities develop. The previously supple deformities are no longer correctable with manipulation and become static deformities.[9] Typically, the clinical picture of spastic cerebral palsy that most commonly affects the foot and ankle is overactive ankle plantar flexors and ineffective dorsiflexors, although exact presentation varies.[4,9]

CLINICAL COURSE

After an insult to the central nervous system, it can take days to weeks for spasticity to develop.[4,6] Following an acute injury, there is often a brief period of flaccid paralysis and hypotonia. Deep tendon reflexes are also diminished during this time, which can last from a few hours to weeks.[6,8] Elevated muscle tone and hyperreflexia then develop, although this is followed by a long period of spontaneous recovery. During this time, spasticity can improve with the return of strength, coordination, and sensation. Cognitive function also improves throughout this period, as a new baseline is established. Following CVA, recovery continues for 6 to 9 months, whereas TBIs continue to improve for about 18 months.[2,6] Recognition of the duration and spontaneous recovery potential is important for evaluation and surgical planning.

Initially, spastic-type cerebral palsy also presents with hypotonia and weakness, which progresses to hypertonia and spasticity.[4] Patients have pain with ambulation, shoe wear, and use of orthotic devices and demonstrate combinations of tripping, in-toeing, and out-toeing.[9]

CLINICAL CONDITIONS

Spastic equinovarus is the most common foot and ankle deformity both following CVA[2,3] and also in cerebral palsy (**Fig. 1**).[10] It usually results from spasticity of the plantarflexor and invertor muscles, combined with a deficiency of their associated antagonists.[2] Specifically, spasticity can be seen in a combination of several different muscles including gastrocnemius, soleus, anterior tibialis, posterior tibialis, flexor hallucis longus (FHL), and flexor digitorum longus (FDL), while associated weakness can be seen in the peroneals.[4,5,8,9,11–13] In TBI and CVA patients, varus is typically caused by spasticity of tibialis anterior, whereas tibialis posterior often produces the deformity

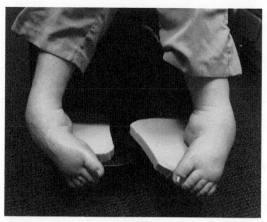

Fig. 1. Marked spastic equinovarus deformity secondary to progressive brain disorder. Note the varus and supinated forefoot as well as the varus heel, indicating involvement of both the anterior tibialis and the PTTs.

in cerebral palsy.[6,10,12] Clinically, the deforming forces cause equinovarus before and on heel strike. Long-term sequelae of these altered kinetics include lateral callosities and lateral instability during stance.[11]

Marked flexion deformities of the toes are frequently seen due to overactivity of both the long and the short toe flexors (**Fig. 2**). This condition worsens with correction of the equinus position of the ankle. Paradoxically, sometimes spasticity of the extensor

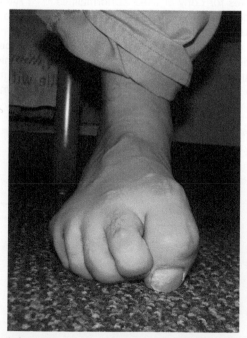

Fig. 2. Severe flexion deformities of the toes secondary to CVA. Note the deformity at both the PIP and the DIP joints indicating involvement of both the short and the long toe flexor tendons.

hallucis longus (EHL) contributes to the varus foot position, which is noted by hyper-extension of the hallux (**Fig. 3**).

Spastic equinovalgus is an alternative deformity seen in cerebral palsy, which can be very difficult to manage given the intense pull of the triceps surae and tarsal collapse (**Fig. 4**).[10] This deformity is secondary to spasticity of the plantarflexors and evertors of the foot. In addition, hallux valgus can develop secondary to imbalance between the intrinsic and extrinsic muscles of the foot (abductor and adductor hallucis, EHL) or the planovalgus foot position and resultant pressure on the medial aspect of the hallux.

CLINICAL EVALUATION

Physical examination of foot and ankle deformities should be thorough. Observational gait analysis must be from the front, side, and back, evaluating foot position in each phase of gait.[9,12] The Functional Ambulation Classification classifies patients into 6 groups based on level of ambulation (**Table 1**).[14] Evidence of atypical shoe wear can indicate disrupted loading patterns.[9] On skin examination, one should evaluate for calluses commonly seen on the lateral plantar foot and tips of toes. Special attention should also be paid to areas of possible ulceration, especially in the setting of contractures, including toe creases, hindfoot, knee and popliteal fossa, lateral hip, and groin.[6] Standing examination should evaluate hindfoot alignment, arch height (presence of midfoot collapse, pronation, or supination), and forefoot deformities, such as hammer toes, claw toes, or hallux valgus.[7] Alignment examination must be performed in both weight-bearing and non-weight-bearing conditions.[9] Passive range of motion of the ankle, hindfoot, midfoot, and forefoot determines the flexibility of deformities and evaluates for bony or fixed abnormalities.[6,7,12] Although it still can be useful and should be done, the Silfverskiold test may not be accurate in patients with spasticity.[10] Muscle tone, deep tendon reflexes, evaluation for ankle or hallux clonus, and degree of rigidity should be recorded. Tone may be graded using the Modified Ashworth Scale (**Table 2**).[15] On motor and strength examination, quantitative evaluation with dynamometry may be useful.[6] Sensation may be impaired after TBI or CVA, although pain may persist from conditions, such as complex regional pain

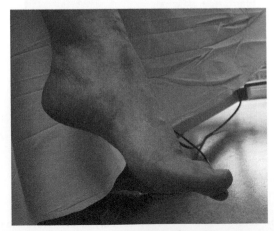

Fig. 3. Hyperextension of the hallux in a mild case of spastic equinovarus, indicating over-activity of the EHL.

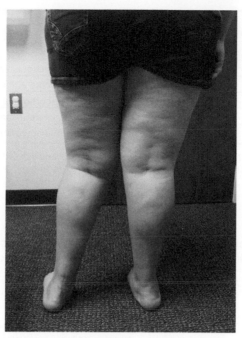

Fig. 4. Spastic equinovalgus ankle deformity in an adult cerebral palsy patient. Note the posterior scar indicating previous Achilles lengthening procedure.

syndrome, muscle tension, heterotopic ossification, occult fractures, or peripheral neuropathy, and should be noted. A standard vascular examination is especially important in stroke patients, given the shared risk factors between vascular disease and CVA.[1]

One of the most useful diagnostic studies available for preoperative planning is dynamic electromyogram (EMG).[9,11,12,16,17] In a dynamic EMG, muscle activity and pattern are recorded during ambulation to allow distinction between normal phasic activity, spastic, nonphasic activity, or paralytic activity.[6,7,9,12] Muscles tested include anterior tibialis, posterior tibialis, gastrocnemius, soleus, flexor hallucis longus, flexor digitorum longus, peroneus longus, and peroneus brevis.[18] In normal gait, the tibialis anterior should be active in eccentric contraction during initial contact and loading and then again in concentric contraction during mid- to late-swing phase. Quiescence is expected between the 2 phases. Fifty percent of TBI patients have been reported as showing continuous activity in tibialis anterior throughout gait.[12] Examining 41 spastic equinovarus deformities, Fuller and colleagues[8] showed that supplementing a thorough clinical evaluation with preoperative instrumented gait analysis, with dynamic EMG as a component, resulted in alteration of 64% of the predetermined surgical plans and increased intersurgeon agreement to a significant degree.[8]

Standard weight-bearing radiographic series of the foot and ankle should also be obtained to evaluate for bony anomalies, although in severe cases weight-bearing may not be possible. Cavus deformities are common in this condition, which is particularly noted on the lateral foot radiograph in either the hindfoot (increased calcaneal pitch), midfoot (apex dorsal talo-first metatarsal angle), or both.[7,19] The varus component of the deformity is noted with significant adduction at the talonavicular joint, or "overcoverage" of the navicular on the talar head (**Fig. 5**).

Table 1 Functional ambulation scale	
0	Nonambulatory
1	Nonfunctional ambulation
2	Household ambulation
3	Neighborhood ambulation
4	Independent community ambulation
5	Normal ambulation

Adapted from Viosca E, Martinez JL, Almagro PL, et al. Proposal and validation of a new functional ambulation classification scale for clinical use. Arch Phys Med Rehabil 2005;86(6):1234–8; with permission.

TREATMENT

Dynamic EMG has showed no difference in the deforming muscular forces causing spastic deformities in patients with TBI and CVA. Hence they can be treated in a similar fashion.[18]

Nonoperative

Early management focuses on preventing deformity with orthotic bracing.[3,4,6] During the period of spontaneous recovery, physical therapy and bracing attempt to maintain joint motion and prevent contractures. Muscle weakness is more amenable to bracing, and dynamic splinting and traction should be used with caution, as these may increase spasticity or clonus.[6] A rigid ankle foot orthosis (AFO) is useful for flexible spastic foot drop, providing foot and ankle flexibility, foot clearance, improved knee control, and a more balanced gait.[7] Serial casting, in which soft tissue is slowly stretched and gradually corrected with weekly cast changes, can be effective in children, especially when the goal is to delay surgery until skeletal maturity. Muscle relaxants, such as baclofen, diazepam, and dantrolene, can augment serial casting or orthotic use, although their effectiveness can be limited by side effects.[6]

Local anesthetic nerve blocks may be beneficial to temporarily remove spasticity during serial casting and should be placed with the aid of a nerve stimulator.[6,7] Phenol nerve blocks with a 3% to 5% solution may decrease spasticity for several months and should be used within the early phase of CVA and TBI, at 6 and 18 months,

Table 2 Modified Ashworth scale (spasticity grade)	
0	No increase in muscle tone throughout flexion/extension
1	Slight increase in muscle tone (catch/release at end of range of motion)
1+	Slight increase in muscle tone (catch and minimal resistance throughout <50% range of motion)
2	Marked increase in muscle tone through most of range of motion but passive motion easy
3	Considerable increase in muscle tone with difficult passive motion
4	Rigid in flexion/extension

Reprinted from Phys Ther 1987;67(2):206–7, with permission of the American Physical Therapy Association. Copyright 1987 American Physical Therapy Association.

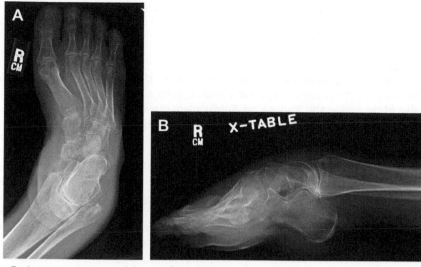

Fig. 5. Anteroposterior and lateral foot radiograph in a patient with severe equinovarus. Note the overcoverage at the talonavicular joint (*A*) and the significant midfoot equinus (*B*).

respectively. Open blocks generally show greater efficacy and duration than when administered blindly, secondary to more accurate placement.[6] Botulinum toxin injection can reduce muscular tone, improve gait, and reduce aberrant muscle activation. Although efficacy generally decreases with repeated usage, an advantage over nerve injections is that injection does not require precise placement.[4,6,7]

Electrical stimulation has been used after the acute phase to help retain strength and has been shown to increase dorsiflexion and decrease spastic reflexes. Peroneal nerve stimulation has been shown to improve inversion and symmetry of gait.[7]

Operative

Indications for surgery include deformities that do not respond to multidisciplinary nonoperative approaches. Patients should be at a plateau of neurologic improvement, which is typically 6 months following CVA and 18 months following TBI.[6,18] Namdari and colleagues[2] investigated outcomes of split anterior tibialis tendon transfer (SPLATT) in a cohort of stroke patients with spastic equinovarus deformities and reported age and sex did not affect outcomes and all patients had improvement despite a wide range of elapsed time since their stroke.[2] Wheelchair-bound patients are not excluded from surgery if the correction will produce a plantigrade foot that can more easily be placed on a wheelchair foot platform.[6] Specific goals of surgery are a balanced, functional foot, minimization of bracing, pain relief, callus and ulcer prevention, facilitated hygiene, and allowance for positioning in a wheelchair.[2,6,9,11,12]

Early in the course of spastic foot and ankle deformities, the deformity is dynamic and should generally be treated by balancing muscles with lengthening or transfer. Although static deformities have fixed capsules, ligaments, muscles, and/or tendons, these may be treated as dynamic deformities after releasing the spastic structures. Differentiating between a dynamic and static deformity can be difficult, especially in the clinic setting. A thorough intraoperative evaluation while the patient is under anesthesia that is compared with the preoperative evaluation can help to determine whether the deformity is dynamic or static. Longstanding static deformities can become a bony deformity, which then requires osteotomies in addition to muscle balancing. Arthrodesis is reserved for severe or revision cases and can improve the shape of the foot at the expense of shock absorption.[4,9]

Equinus deformity

Tendo achilles and gastrocnemius-soleus lengthening If the equinus deformity does not correct once the patient is under anesthesia, then a static contracture is present that should be addressed through an Achilles lengthening. However, if the equinus deformity does correct with anesthesia, a primarily dynamic deformity is present that should respond to proximal lengthening. One must be very careful not to over-lengthen and cause a calcaneal gait.[6,12]

The most common procedure performed for an Achilles contracture is a percutaneous triple hemisection tenotomy (Hoke lengthening).[6,9] In this procedure, transverse hemisections of the Achilles tendon are performed through 3 stab incisions starting in the midline while the foot is held in maximum dorsiflexion. Generally (for a varus deformity) the most distal and proximal incisions address the medial half of the Achilles, while the middle incision addresses the lateral half of the Achilles. The orientation of the hemisection can be reversed for a valgus deformity (**Fig. 6**).[6,12,20] Alternatively, an open Z-lengthening using an 8-cm incision medial to the Achilles tendon may be performed. In severe longstanding cases with associated joint contractures, a dynamic thin-wire external fixation device can be used to achieve equinus correction in combination with the soft tissue procedures discussed in the following section on Varus Deformity (**Fig. 7**).[21]

If the deformity is determined to be primarily dynamic, a proximal gastrocnemius and soleus lengthening should be performed. In this procedure the junction between the gastrocnemius and soleus muscle bellies is identified in the midleg from a medial approach. The individual tendons overlying the respective muscle bellies are then transected and lengthened along the muscle belly with dorsiflexion of the foot.[20] These procedures are generally performed in conjunction with other procedures, which then dictate the postoperative course.

Calf weakness Calf weakness in patients with spastic equinovarus deformity may result from the inherent weakness of spastic muscles or as a result of surgical

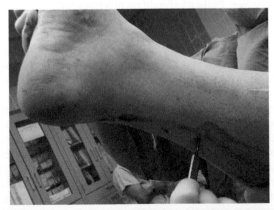

Fig. 6. Triple hemisection Achilles tenotomy (Hoke lengthening). The blade is inserted longitudinally in the midline of the Achilles and turned 90°, and then the hand is raised to perform a transverse cut of either the medial or the lateral half of the Achilles tendon at the appropriate level.

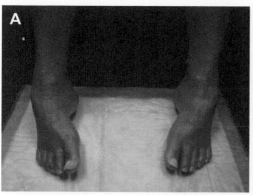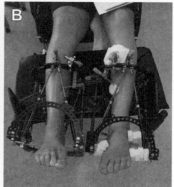

Fig. 7. Spastic equinovarus feet secondary to severe Guillain-Barre disease (*A*). Clinical photo-graph (midcorrection on *right*, first postoperative visit on *left*) after TAL, posteromedial release including PTT lengthening, and dynamic thin-wire external fixation placement (*B*).

treatment to correct the equinus deformity. Although a tendoachilles lengthening or proximal gastrocnemius-soleus lengthening corrects equinus, it does so at the cost of weakening the gastrocnemius-soleus complex. Calf weakness contributes to the frequent necessity of postoperative orthoses. To decrease the likelihood of continuing to require an ankle-foot-orthosis, transfers of the FHL or FDL tendon to the os calcis may be used. Transferring the FDL tendon has been described for spastic equinovarus patients using a 3-incision technique with good results.[17,20] Thirty-nine percent of pa-tients treated this way only required an orthotic postoperatively as opposed to 69% treated without FHL or FDL transfer. Of note, 2 of 30 of such patients had mild correctable equines, which did not require further orthotics.[17] The authors prefer to use an FHL tendon transfer through a single-incision technique to avoid the potential for neurovascular compromise as the FDL transfer must cross the neurovascular bundle. The FHL is harvested through an incision just medial to the distal Achilles tendon and is transected as far distal as possible within its fibro-osseous tunnel. The FHL can then be secured to the os calcis just anterior to the insertion of the Achil-les using a bioabsorbable interference screw.[22,23]

Varus deformity
SPLATT The varus component of the equinovarus deformity is most commonly sec-ondary to an overactive tibialis anterior muscle. Therefore a common and useful pro-cedure to correct this portion of the deformity is a SPLATT. In this procedure the lateral half of the anterior tibialis tendon is transferred to the cuboid or lateral cunei-form to balance the foot in a neutral position. Originally devised by Garett and described by Hoffer for cerebral palsy, its indications have expanded to include any spastic varus or equinovarus deformity.[12,24] This procedure is indicated when there is dynamic varus or equinovarus in a patient over 4 years of age.[12] It is often done in combination with a TAL and is one of the most common and successful tendon transfers known to orthopedic surgery.[6,7,12,20] A 3-incision technique is used (**Fig. 8**). First, a medial incision overlying the insertion of the anterior tibialis on the medial cuneiform is performed. The lateral half of the anterior tibialis tendon is split longitudinally and transected at its insertion as far distal as possible. The second inci-sion is made 8 to 10 cm proximal to the ankle joint just lateral to the tibial crest. The fascia overlying the tibialis anterior is divided and the lateral half of the tendon is passed from distal to proximal. The final incision is placed over the cuboid or lateral

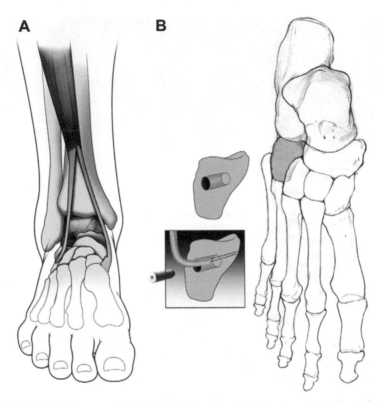

Fig. 8. SPLATT. (*A*) The completed SPLATT transfer. (*B*) The tunnel in the cuboid bone for the lateral arm of the tibialis anterior tendon. (*From* Keenan MA. The management of spastic equinovarus deformity following stroke and head injury. Foot Ankle Clin 2011;16(3):499–514; with permission.)

cuneiform, and the tendon is redirected in a subcutaneous fashion from proximal to distal. A bone tunnel is then created perpendicular to the surface and the tendon is passed and secured with an interference screw.[6,12,25] It has been suggested that a lateromedial (starting point perpendicular to the bone surface) routing is superior to traditional plantar-dorsal routing and proven to have stronger pullout strength and a longer bony canal. Interference screw fixation has demonstrated strength to failure of 166N, 44N stronger than traditional fixation.[5] It is important to balance the tension of the transferred portion of the tibialis anterior with the medial intact portion with the foot in a neutral position to avoid overcorrection or undercorrection. However some authors advocate for transfer of the entire anterior tibialis tendon and a cadaver study has demonstrated neither split nor whole tendon transfer led to overcorrection (**Fig. 9**).[26,27] If bone quality is poor, the tendon can be tenodesed to the peroneus brevis tendon near its insertion.

Postoperatively, a short leg cast or splint is placed before reversal of anesthesia to hold the foot in a corrected position. A walking cast is applied at 2 weeks postoperatively and transitioned to either a walking boot or an AFO at 6 weeks for an additional 6 weeks. Longer-term AFO use may be required depending on the rehabilitation of the patient and maintenance of a plantigrade foot. Passive plantarflexion should be avoided.

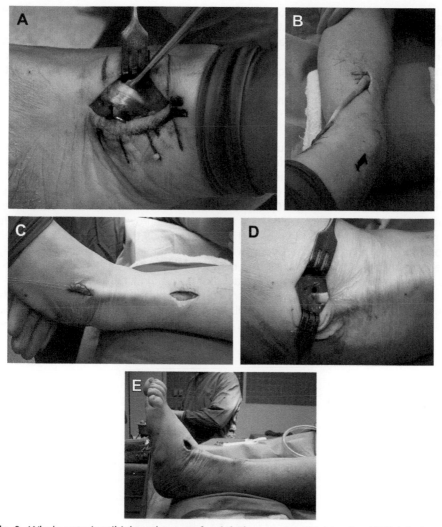

Fig. 9. Whole anterior tibial tendon transfer. (*A*) The anterior tibial tendon (ATT) is isolated from the insertion on the medial cuneiform. (*B*) The tendon is harvested about 10 cm proximal to the ankle joint. (*C*) The tendon is passed in a subcutaneous fashion from proximal to distal, exiting at an incision overlying the lateral cuneiform. (*D*) Insertion of the tendon into the lateral cuneiform using a bioabsorbable interference screw. (*E*) Corrected stance of the foot after transfer.

Long toe flexor (FHL/FDL) transfer Alternatively, the long toe flexors (FHL and FDL) have been transferred through the interosseous membrane as an alternative to the SPLATT procedure for spastic equinovarus with good success.[28–30] This procedure generally requires a long harvest of the toe flexor tendons from the midfoot, transfer from posterior to anterior through the interosseous membrane, and tenodesing to the anterior toe extensors or inserted into the cuneiforms.

Fractional lengthening of posterior tibialis tendon Fractional lengthening of the posterior tibialis tendon (PTT) is indicated when dynamic EMG shows continuous activity in this muscle, which is most common in cerebral palsy. Some spastic CVA and TBI patients also have a component of PTT spasticity that contributes to hindfoot varus, although in general the tibialis anterior spasticity dominates. To achieve a fractional lengthening, an incision is made 4 cm above the medial malleolus posterior to the tibia. The myotendinous junction is incised with 2 to 3 incisions a few centimeters apart with manipulation of the foot to achieve correction. This incision is often performed in conjunction with and before performing the SPLATT procedure.[6,12]

Toe deformities

Hyperextension of the hallux due to overactivity of the EHL is an underappreciated deformity in spastic equinovarus patients.[20] This spasticity can also contribute to the varus foot deformity. When the hyperextended hallux is symptomatic, transferring the EHL tendon to the dorsum of the foot can correct this problem as well as aid in ankle dorsiflexion force (**Fig. 10**) and is usually achieved through an incision over the middle cuneiform while taking care to avoid the neurovascular bundle. The EHL tendon is transected, and the proximal tendon stump is then transferred through a bone tunnel in the middle cuneiform with interference screw fixation as previously described while holding the ankle at a neutral position. The distal stump is sutured to the extensor digitorum brevis or the anterior tibialis tendon.

Flexion deformities of the toes are very common in spastic equinovarus deformity because of overactivity of the FHL, FDL, and their associated brevis muscles. This spasticity can also contribute to the equinus aspect of the deformity, with the toe

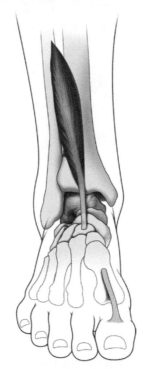

Fig. 10. The transfer of the EHL tendon to the middle cuneiform bone. (*From* Keenan MA. The management of spastic equinovarus deformity following stroke and head injury. Foot Ankle Clin 2011;16(3):499–514.)

deformity unmasked or accentuated when the equinovarus position is corrected. Plantar 2-cm longitudinal incisions are made over the proximal flexion creases. The tendon sheaths are opened, and both the short- and the long-flexor tendons are transected sharply using a scalpel.[6,12,31] Retrograde pinning of the toes for 4 weeks can be considered if there is concern for recurrence.

Equinovalgus and hallux valgus deformities

Spastic equinoplanovalgus deformities are most commonly seen in the cerebral palsy patient and may be addressed during childhood. This deformity is generally caused by overactivity of the plantarflexors (gastrocnemius-soleus complex) and evertor (peroneals) muscle groups. Moderate deformities that do not respond to botulinum injection may be corrected with a peroneus brevis to longus transfer with a TAL. More severe deformities with bony anomalies can generally be corrected by a peroneus brevis to longus transfer combined with a TAL and lateral column lengthening through the anterior process of the calcaneus.[9] Revision cases may require TAL and either subtalar or possibly triple arthrodesis.[32] Hallux valgus rarely occurs in isolation and is generally a result of equinovalgus. Specific treatment of the hallux valgus deformity is beyond the scope of this article but should focus on traditional osteotomies for deformity correction versus arthrodesis of the first metatarsophalangeal joint given the neuromuscular cause.[9]

Fixed deformities

Severe and chronic fixed varus hindfoot deformities can result from a longstanding spastic condition more commonly in the younger patient with a developing skeleton. These patients usually have some degree of varus at the subtalar joint and secondary medial soft tissue contraction. Associated midfoot equinus and adduction is common and very important to recognize. In this situation, soft tissue procedures alone will not correct the fixed bone deformity. Subtalar arthrodesis and/or midfoot osteotomy may be required to address the different components of the deformity. The appropriate soft tissue procedures previously described should be considered in combination with the bone correction, in particular, a TAL, tibialis posterior lengthening with talonavicular joint capsule and spring ligament release, and possibly SPLATT to help with dorsiflexion. The subtalar arthrodesis should be performed through a standard sinus tarsi incision. In severe deformities a closing wedge can be performed through the joint by resecting bone from the lateral aspect of both the talus and the calcaneus. Standard screw fixation should be used. Alternatively, lateralizing calcaneal osteotomy of the tuberosity with or without a closing wedge may be performed.[6] In severe cases, gradual correction with a thin-wire external fixation device can be a useful tool to address both the ankle and the foot deformities simultaneously.

RESULTS AND OUTCOMES

Surgical intervention for spastic equinovarus deformity has been shown to be an effective treatment to achieve the primary goals of a balanced, functional foot with minimization of bracing and reduced pain. Patients improve their ambulatory function as well as decrease the need for orthotics and assistive devices following correction.[2,11,13,18] In addition, earlier operative intervention may be more cost-effective than continued nonoperative care due to a decrease in the use of physical therapy and orthotics. Reddy and colleagues[3] showed that 19 of 29 patients discontinued physical therapy after surgical correction and 17 (58.6%) discontinued the used of orthotics. One recent study with a short mean follow-up (50 weeks) showed 44% of patients were brace-free and 48% were free of ambulatory assistive devices.[2] In a study by Keenan and colleagues[18] with longer-term follow-up (50 months), 31% of patients were brace-free following SPLATT with 60% of nonambulators becoming ambulators. Morita and colleagues[29] reported better results with a long toe flexor transfer (75% brace-free) compared with anterior tibial tendon transfer (53% brace-free) at a minimum 2-year follow-up. In addition, 15% of patients in both groups had recurrence of the varus deformity. In a large study with 84 feet available for follow-up, 80 of 82 patients were satisfied and would recommend surgery to another patient and their functional autonomy increased by an average of one level.[13] It has been noted that TBI patients and nonambulators have worse outcomes, which may be secondary to the severity of their deformities and sensory deficits.[11]

SUMMARY

Spastic foot and ankle deformities are the result of numerous central nervous system pathologic abnormalities that can be severely debilitating to affected patients. The most important preoperative evaluation is with a dynamic EMG, which can drastically influence the way these deformities are approached. Surgery should be considered when nonoperative treatments are no longer effective and the patient's condition is no longer improving. The specific surgical intervention should be tailored to the patient's specific deformity, with many patients having multiple components to their deformity. The most common procedures performed are the SPLATT and lengthening of the Achilles tendon or gastrocsoleus complex caused by the frequency of anterior tibialis spasticity and associated equinus contracture. Often orthotic devices can often be discontinued and ambulation levels increase predictably following surgical correction.

REFERENCES

1. Go AS, Mozaffarian D, Roger VL, et al. Heart disease and stroke statistics–2013 update: a report from the American Heart Association. Circulation 2013;127(1): e6–245.
2. Namdari S, Park MJ, Baldwin K, et al. Effect of age, sex, and timing on correction of spastic equinovarus following cerebrovascular accident. Foot Ankle Int 2009; 30(10):923–7.
3. Reddy S, Kusuma S, Hosalkar H, et al. Surgery can reduce the nonoperative care associated with an equinovarus foot deformity. Clin Orthop Relat Res 2008; 466(7):1683–7.
4. Woods RJ, Cervone RL, Fernandez HH. Common neurologic disorders affecting the foot. J Am Podiatr Med Assoc 2004;94(2):104–17.
5. Hosalkar H, Goebel J, Reddy S, et al. Fixation techniques for split anterior tibialis transfer in spastic equinovarus feet. Clin Orthop Relat Res 2008;466(10):2500–6.
6. Botte MJ, Bruffey JD, Copp SN, et al. Surgical reconstruction of acquired spastic foot and ankle deformity. Foot Ankle Clin 2000;5(2):381–416.
7. Strauss NE, Angell DK. Foot conditions related to neuromuscular disorders in adults. Phys Med Rehabil 2001;15(3):489–500.
8. Fuller DA, Keenan MA, Esquenazi A, et al. The impact of instrumented gait analysis on surgical planning: treatment of spastic equinovarus deformity of the foot and ankle. Foot Ankle Int 2002;23(8):738–43.
9. Davids JR. The foot and ankle in cerebral palsy. Orthop Clin North Am 2010; 41(4):579–93.
10. Vogler HW. Surgical management of neuromuscular deformities of the foot and ankle in children and adolescents. Clin Podiatr Med Surg 1987;4(1):175–206.

11. Edwards P, Hsu J. SPLATT combined with tendo achilles lengthening for spastic equinovarus in adults: results and predictors of surgical outcome. Foot Ankle 1993;14(6):335–8.

12. Piccioni L, Keenan ME. Surgical correction of varus and equinovarus deformity in the spastic patient. Oper Tech Orthop 1992;2(3):146–50.

13. Vogt JC, Bach G, Cantini B, et al. Split anterior tibial tendon transfer for varus equinus spastic foot deformity initial clinical findings correlate with functional results: a series of 132 operated feet. Foot Ankle Surg 2011;17(3):178–81.

14. Viosca E, Martinez JL, Almagro PL, et al. Proposal and validation of a new functional ambulation classification scale for clinical use. Arch Phys Med Rehabil 2005;86(6):1234–8.

15. Bohannon RW, Smith MB. Interrater reliability of a modified Ashworth scale of muscle spasticity. Phys Ther 1987;67(2):206–7.

16. Jordan C. Current status of functional lower extremity surgery in adult spastic patients. Clin Orthop Relat Res 1988;(233):102–9.

17. Keenan MA, Lee GA, Tuckman AS, et al. Improving calf muscle strength in patients with spastic equinovarus deformity by transfer of the long toe flexors to the Os calcis. J Head Trauma Rehabil 1999;14(2):163–75.

18. Keenan MA, Creighton J, Garland DE, et al. Surgical correction of spastic equinovarus deformity in the adult head trauma patient. Foot Ankle 1984;5(1):35–41.

19. Klammer G, Benninger E, Espinosa N. The varus ankle and instability. Foot Ankle Clin 2012;17(1):57–82.

20. Keenan MA. The management of spastic equinovarus deformity following stroke and head injury. Foot Ankle Clin 2011;16(3):499–514.

21. Cuttica DJ, Decarbo WT, Philbin TM. Correction of rigid equinovarus deformity using a multiplanar external fixator. Foot Ankle Int 2011;32(5):S533–9.

22. Den Hartog BD. Flexor hallucis longus transfer for chronic Achilles tendonosis. Foot Ankle Int 2003;24(3):233–7.

23. Elias I, Raikin SM, Besser MP, et al. Outcomes of chronic insertional Achilles tendinosis using FHL autograft through single incision. Foot Ankle Int 2009;30(3):197–204.

24. Hoffer MM, Garrett A, Brink J, et al. The orthopaedic management of brain injured children. J Bone Joint Surg Am 1971;53A:567–76.

25. Fuller DA, McCarthy JJ, Keenan MA. The use of the absorbable interference screw for a split anterior tibial tendon (SPLATT) transfer procedure. Orthopedics 2004;27(4):372–4.

26. Henderson CP, Parks BG, Guyton GP. Lateral and medial plantar pressures after split versus whole anterior tibialis tendon transfer. Foot Ankle Int 2008;29(10):1038–41.

27. Pinzur MS, Sherman R, DiMonte-Levine P, et al. Adult-onset hemiplegia: changes in gait after muscle-balancing procedures to correct the equinus deformity. J Bone Joint Surg Am 1986;68(8):1249–57.

28. Bibbo C, Jaglan SS. Tendon transfers for equinovarus deformity in adults and children. Foot Ankle Clin 2011;16(3):401–18.

29. Morita S, Muneta T, Yamamoto H, et al. Tendon transfer for equinovarus deformed foot caused by cerebrovascular disease. Clin Orthop Relat Res 1998;(350):166–73.

30. Ono K, Hiroshima K, Tada K, et al. Anterior transfer of the toe flexors for equinovarus deformity of the foot. Int Orthop 1980;4(3):225–9.

31. Keenan MA, Gorai AP, Smith CW, et al. Intrinsic toe flexion deformity following correction of spastic equinovarus deformity in adults. Foot Ankle 1987;7(6):333–7.

32. Banks HH. The management of spastic deformities of the foot and ankle. Clin Orthop Relat Res 1977;(122):70–6.

Percutaneous Techniques for Tendon Transfers in the Foot and Ankle

Vinod Kumar Panchbhavi, MD

KEYWORDS

- Achilles tendon • Posterior tibial tendon dysfunction • Flexor hallucis longus tendon
- Flexor digitorum longus • Chronic tear • Tendinopathy

KEY POINTS

- The plantar approach is a minimally invasive approach to the medial approach to locate and harvest long flexor tendons.
- A connecting band between the long flexor tendons needs division if present.
- The neurovascular structures can be visualized directly through the plantar approach and can be retracted safely.
- The plantar skin incision is in a relatively nonweight-bearing part of the foot and tolerated well.

INTRODUCTION

The conditions in which tendon transfer techniques are frequently utilized include posterior tibial tendon and Achilles tendon disorders. Flexor digitorum longus (FDL) tendon in the vicinity is transferred to the navicular bone to reconstruct the posterior tibial tendon, and flexor hallucis longus (FHL) tendon is transferred to the calcaneus to reconstruct the Achilles tendon.

The surgical technique to harvest FDL tendon was described by Mann and Thompson.[1] They advocated a medial-based approach and a dissection that proceeded along the FDL tendon in the deeper layers from the medial border of the foot toward the midfoot laterally.

A similar open approach was reported by Wapner and colleagues[2] for harvesting the FHL tendon. This approach required an incision placed on the medial border of the midfoot, extending from the navicular tuberosity to the head of the first metatarsal when FHL was used for reconstruction of chronic tears of the Achilles tendon.

These open medial approaches to harvesting the FDL and FHL, however, require an incision that extends along almost the entire medial border of the foot and an

Department of Orthopedic Surgery, University of Texas Medical Branch, Galveston, TX 77555-0165, USA
E-mail address: vkpanchb@utmb.edu

Foot Ankle Clin N Am 19 (2014) 113–122
http://dx.doi.org/10.1016/j.fcl.2013.10.008
1083-7515/14/$ – see front matter © 2014 Elsevier Inc. All rights reserved.

foot.theclinics.com

extensive, deep, and difficult dissection. The dissection starts from the incision and is carried across the midfoot in the vicinity of blood vessels and nerves almost to the midfoot to reach the tendons in the depth of the surgical exposure. There is a risk for injury to the medial and lateral plantar neurovascular structures.[3–5] A longer incision and longer exposure are required because of an indirect approach to the point of division of the tendon (**Figs. 1** and **2**).

This article describes percutaneous techniques to harvest the FHL and FDL tendons through small incisions placed directly overlying the tendon in the midfoot and forefoot.

INDICATIONS

An FDL tendon transfer is indicated in patients who have failed conservative management for posterior tibial tendon dysfunction and in cases in which the tendon is found to be severely degenerated or beyond repair.

An FHL tendon transfer is indicated in patients with chronic rupture of the Achilles tendon who remain symptomatic with poor function in whom operative repair is being considered. End-to-end repair is possible for Achilles tendon defects less than 2 cm, and V-Y advancement of the Achilles tendon can bridge defects ranging 2 to 6 cm long. In gaps over 6 cm long, however, adjacent tendons such as the FHL tendon can be transferred to the calcaneus to provide plantar flexion at ankle.[6]

CONTRAINDICATIONS

Operative intervention is contraindicated in patients with poor wound healing potential, including patients with peripheral vascular disease, poor soft tissue envelope, chronic venous or lymph stasis, and peripheral neuropathy. In a competitive athlete requiring normal great toe function, use of the FHL tendon can affect performance; therefore, an alternative technique is preferred in this situation.

PREOPERATIVE PLANNING

The neurovascular status and condition of soft tissues in the leg and the foot should be evaluated and documented. The FHL and FDL frequently have interconnections in the midfoot. The presence of these interconnections can be determined preoperatively. Flexion of the lesser toes when the great toe is being actively flexed or vice versa is indicative of the presence of an interconnecting band between the FDL and FHL tendons. Patients are counseled regarding possible weakness in plantar flexion in the

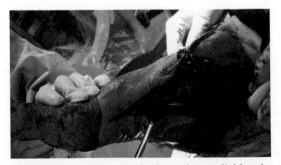

Fig. 1. An open surgical exposure that extends along the medial border of the foot undertaken to follow the FDL tendon into the midfoot for harvesting and transfer to navicular bone in a patient with posterior tibial tendon dysfunction.

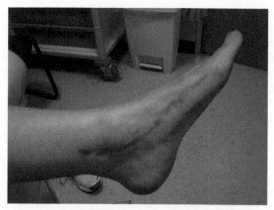

Fig. 2. A resultant long scar from a procedure as described in **Fig. 1**.

toes. A likely deficit in great toe flexion power and its effect on athletic activity should be mentioned when reconstruction of the ruptured Achilles tendon is contemplated using the FHL tendon.

SURGICAL TECHNIQUE
FDL Tendon Harvest Technique

Preparation
The FDL tendon for posterior tibial tendon reconstruction is harvested with the patient in the supine position. A thigh tourniquet is applied in preference to a calf tourniquet. A calf tourniquet can tether muscle bellies and interfere with the determination of appropriate musculotendinous length and tension in the tendon transferred. A single dose of an antibiotic is administered intravenously for prophylaxis against infection.

- The location where the FDL starts dividing into individual slips for the lesser toes can be determined on the plantar surface of the foot using the coordinates previously described by Panchbhavi and colleagues.[7] The authors described that the FDL division was located topographically on the plantar surface of the foot, approximately midway between the back of the heel and the base of the second toe and at this midpoint, about two-thirds of the width medially from the lateral border of the foot.
- A metallic ruler is held parallel to the plantar surface of the foot and a line drawn from the back of the heel to the proximal flexor crease at the base of the second toe and the midpoint marked. Another line is drawn at this midpoint perpendicular to the previous vertical line. A point two-thirds of the distance away from the lateral border of the foot on this second line marks the location of the FDL division. A vertical skin marking about 2 cm long at this second point is used for percutaneous approach to the FDL.
- Additional confirmation for location of plantar incision can be obtained as follows. The sheath of the FDL tendon is identified in the region of the hindfoot through the exposure that is used for the concomitant procedure, such as the exploration of the posterior tibial tendon. A malleable probe with an olive tip, such as the Emmett probe (Cardinal Health, OH, USA), is introduced within the tendon sheath and passed gently distally into the midfoot, where it is easily palpated.
- After the site of the FDL division is located, a vertical incision is made in the plantar skin to expose the central part of the plantar aponeurosis. The vertically

oriented fibers of the aponeurosis are separated to expose the flexor digitorum brevis muscle. The dissection is carried out in the same plane as the incision separating the muscle fibers to expose the FDL tendon. The lateral branch of the medial plantar nerve passes along the medial border of the flexor digitorum brevis and therefore could be at risk. Therefore, it is important to make the plantar incision long enough to allow adequate visualization.

- The identity of the tendon is verified by applying a pulling tension on the tendon through the proximal wound in the hindfoot and assessing transmission of the tension distally to the tendon identified in the midfoot, and at the same time observing maximal flexion either in lesser toes or the great toe.
- The tendon is then cut sharply in the midfoot and the cut end pulled proximally through the wound in the hindfoot region. If there is resistance and if the great toe flexes, a slip between the FDL and FHL tendons exists. Passive plantar flexion of the foot and the toes, as well as pulling distally on the cut end of FDL, brings the interconnection slip into visibility. After this interconnecting band is cut, the resistance is no longer felt, and the FDL tendon can then be pulled proximally for routing into the navicular bone (**Figs. 3** and **4**).

FHL Tendon Harvest Technique

Preparation

The FHL tendon for Achilles tendon reconstruction is harvested with the patient in the prone position. A thigh tourniquet is applied before the patient is turned prone on the operation table. A calf tourniquet is not used. Both lower extremities are prepared from the toes up proximally to a level above the knee and draped to isolate them in a sterile fashion. Draping the uninjured extremity within the sterile field allows direct comparison of the tension imparted to the repaired tendon with that in the intact tendon. A single dose of an antibiotic is administered intravenously for prophylaxis against infection.

The Achilles tendon is approached through a longitudinal incision placed along its medial border. The incision is carried deeper and all the way into the tendon sheath, thus creating full-thickness flaps. The tendon sheath is incised in the line of the incision and reflected off the tendon. The scar tissue in between the ends of the tendon is excised.

If the gap between the cut ends of the tendon is greater than 6 cm, a further procedure of harvesting the FHL tendon is undertaken.

Deeper and medial to the Achilles tendon, the fascia over the posterior compartment and the FHL muscle is identified and incised vertically; the incision is carried distally to expose the tendon of this muscle. A rubber band is looped round the tendon. A pull on the FHL tendon in the hindfoot can be felt in the midfoot and also observed as flexion of the great toe.

The olive tip of a malleable probe similar to one mentioned previously is introduced within the sheath of the FHL tendon and gently passed without resistance distally toward the midfoot. The tip is then palpated in the midfoot. An incision 3 cm in length is made vertically in the plantar aspect of the midfoot. The incision is deepened to expose the plantar fascia. The fibers of the plantar fascia are then separated to expose flexor hallucis brevis muscle. The fibers of this muscle are separated to expose the FHL tendon and the tendon slip that it sends to that branch of the FDL, which goes to the second toe. Deep-bladed retractors are necessary to retract the wound edges and visualize the tendon.

A tendon hook or rubber sling can be passed under the FHL tendon to bring it more superficially into the wound. Similarly, the FDL tendon and the intertendinous slip can

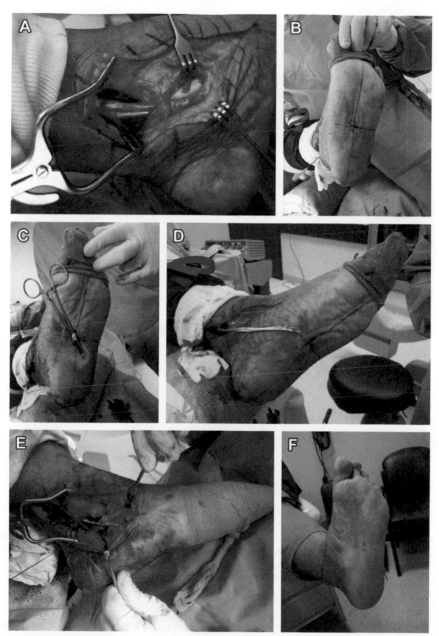

Fig. 3. Intraoperative photographs showing in (*A*) a degenerate posterior tibial tendon and the FDL tendon exposed immediately posterior to the posterior tibial tendon; in (*B*), they show the surface marking used to mark the location of the division of the FDL, reconfirmed by a probe that has been passed through the hindfoot. (*C*) Photograph showing the tendon hooked out. (*D*) Photograph showing the severed FDL tendon brought out through the exposure in the hindfoot. (*E*) Photograph showing the FDL routed through a tunnel in navicular bone. (*F*) A follow-up clinical photograph showing the healed scar in the sole of the foot. The figures also show how a part of the posterior tibial tendon sheath can be retained throughout the operation.

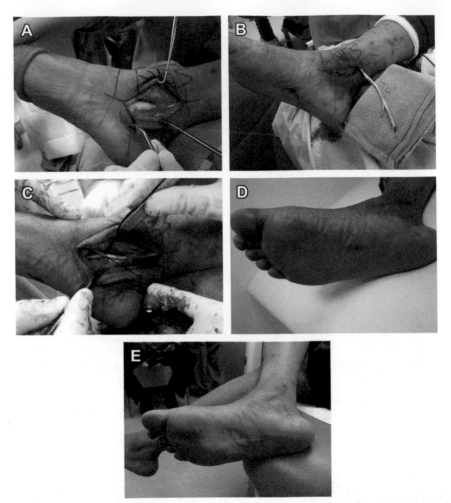

Fig. 4. Intraoperative photographs showing in (*A*) a degenerate posterior tibial tendon; in (*B*), they show the FDL tendon harvested that required severance of a connecting slip seen spread out on the green towel. (*C*) Photograph showing that there is enough length to allow the FDL to be routed through a tunnel in the navicular and to suture it back to itself. (*D*) Photograph showing the plantar scar resulting from the percutaneous harvest at 6 months, (*E*) The same scar barely visible at a 5-year visit for an unrelated reason.

be drawn more superficially into the wound. The tendons can thus be isolated away from the adjacent neurovascular bundle and brought up superficially into the wound to confirm their identity, check for and release intertendinous connections, and perform a safe tenotomy.

The identity of the FHL tendon in the midfoot can be confirmed by pulling the tendon in the hindfoot and checking the transmission of the pull in the midfoot and plantar flexion of the great toe. The tendon can be cut at this level if the length of the graft acquired is deemed adequate for repair. The cut distal stump of the FHL tendon can then be tenodesed to the FDL tendon, holding all toes and the ankle in a neutral position.

When a longer portion of the FHL tendon is required, the FHL tendon is not cut in the midfoot, but more distally at the base of the great toe. A transverse incision 1 cm in length is made in a plantar flexor crease at the base of the great toe. The incision is carried down to the level of the FHL tendon. This tendon is then exposed through its sheath and a rubber band passed to loop around it. The tendon is cut at the base of the great toe. The FHL can then be pulled into the midfoot. Pulling distally on the cut end of FHL brings the interconnection slip between the FHL and FDL tendons into visibility.

After this interconnecting slip is cut, the FHL tendon can be pulled through the wound in the hindfoot and transferred to the calcaneus bone through a transverse tunnel, and the remaining length used to bridge the gap and reconstruct the Achilles tendon (**Fig. 5**).

POSTOPERATIVE MANAGEMENT

The postoperative management following the tendon transfer is tailored by the needs of the concomitant procedures. The limb is rested in a splint to accommodate any swelling, and the wounds are checked at 1 week. A cast replaces the splint, and the tendon transfer is protected for an additional 5 weeks.

A rehabilitation program for strengthening, gait training, and ankle range-of-motion exercises is gradually initiated at 6 weeks, and return to full activities is usually allowed by 12 weeks.

RESULTS

Panchbhavi and colleagues[7] harvested the FDL using the percutaneous technique described in a cadaver study to test the feasibility and safety of this minimally invasive technique. Measurements were obtained to define the location of the division of the FDL tendon in relation to the plantar surface of the foot and the adjacent neurovascular structures. In all of the 83 feet studied, it was possible to harvest the FDL using this technique. In 11 feet (13.25%), a connecting band to the FHL required division. No damage was apparent to the adjacent neurovascular structures on subsequent dissection to expose the underlying layers in the feet. The FDL division was located topographically on the plantar surface of the foot, approximately midway between the back of the heel and the base of the second toe and at this midpoint, about two-thirds of the width medially from the lateral border of the foot. The authors concluded that the FDL tendon can be harvested in the hindfoot after its division through a small plantar incision in the midfoot and that surface anatomy guides placement of the plantar incision over the FDL division.

The author has been using the percutaneous techniques for tendon transfer described here since 2007. The FDL tendon was harvested in 19 cases, and the FHL was harvested in 15 cases. A connecting band between the FDL and FHL tendons required cutting in 31 of the 34 cases. In all cases, the tendons could be successfully harvested through the plantar incision itself, and the length of the harvested tendon was found to be adequate for the primary purpose. There were no instances of intraoperative nerve injury or harvest of a wrong tendon. Postoperatively, 1 patient had hyperesthesia in the midfoot that lasted for 3 months; this had resolved completely by her 6-month checkup.

COMPLICATIONS

Likely complications related to the technique of minimally invasive percutaneous harvesting of the FHL or the FDL tendons include wound infection, wound dehiscence,

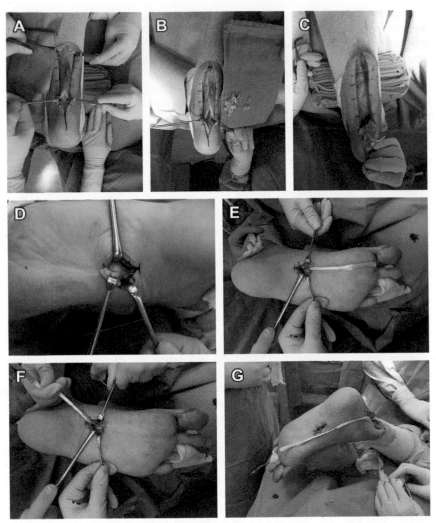

Fig. 5. Intraoperative and follow-up photographs of a patient with chronic degeneration in the Achilles tendon. (*A*) The Achilles tendon exposed at the back of the distal leg. (*B, C*) Photographs show degenerate portions of tendon and calcific bodies excised. (*D*) Photograph shows the sole of the foot with incision overlying and exposing the long flexor tendons. (*E*) Photograph shows the FHL severed through a transverse incision at the base of the great toe and brought out through the exposure in the midfoot. (*F*) Photograph shows the FHL tendon being pulled up to show the connecting band between it and the FDL. (*G*) Photograph shows the FHL brought out through the proximal exposure after severance of the connecting band. (*H–J*) Photographs show the percutaneous incision on the side of the heel used to route the FHL through a transverse tunnel in the calcaneus and the remaining segment of the FHL being used to bridge the gap and reconstruct the Achilles tendon. (*K*) Photograph showing the equal tension and surgical wounds at postoperative follow-up. (*L*) Photograph showing single-limb toe-raise stance on the reconstructed side at a 3-month follow-up.

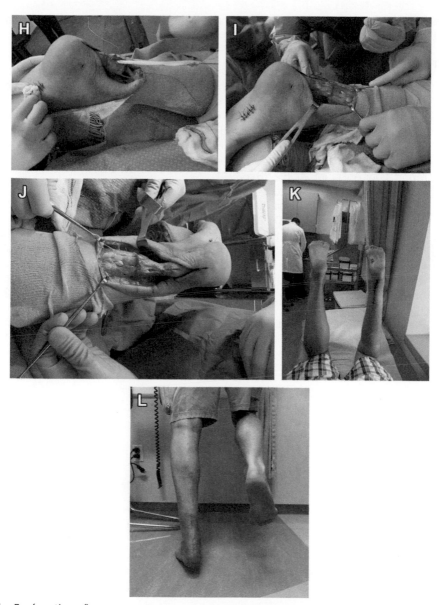

Fig. 5. (*continued*)

painful or hypersensitive plantar scar, medial or lateral plantar nerve or vessel injury, and poor function caused by weakness in plantar flexion of the great toe. These complications, however, are infrequent.

SUMMARY

The percutaneous techniques described here for harvesting the FDL and FHL tendons are minimally invasive alternatives to an open technique or more extensive exposure through the medial border of the foot. The site for dividing the tendons can be more directly approached, and the plantar skin incision's being in a nonweight-bearing part of the foot is well tolerated.

REFERENCES

1. Mann RA, Thompson FM. Rupture of the posterior tibial tendon causing flat foot. Surgical treatment. J Bone Joint Surg Am 1985;67(4):556–61.
2. Wapner KL, Pavlock GS, Hecht PJ, et al. Repair of chronic Achilles tendon rupture with flexor hallucis longus tendon transfer. Foot Ankle 1993;14(8):443–9.
3. Herbst SA, Miller SD. Transection of the medial plantar nerve and hallux cock-up deformity after flexor hallucis longus tendon transfer for Achilles tendonitis: case report. Foot Ankle Int 2006;27(8):639–41.
4. Sullivan RJ, Gladwell HA, Aronow MS, et al. An in vitro study comparing the use of suture anchors and drill hole fixation for flexor digitorum longus transfer to the navicular. Foot Ankle Int 2006;27(5):363–6.
5. Wapner KL, Hecht PJ, Shea JR, et al. Anatomy of second muscular layer of the foot: considerations for tendon selection in transfer for Achilles and posterior tibial tendon reconstruction. Foot Ankle Int 1994;15(8):420–3.
6. Panchbhavi VK. Chronic Achilles tendon repair with flexor hallucis longus tendon harvested using a minimally invasive technique. Tech Foot Ankle Surg 2007;6(2): 123–9.
7. Panchbhavi VK, Yang J, Vallurupalli S. Minimally invasive method of harvesting the flexor digitorum longus tendon: a cadaver study. Foot Ankle Int 2008;29(1): 42–8.

Forefoot Tendon Transfers

Andrea Veljkovic, MD, FRCSC[a,b], Edward Lansang, MD, FRCSC[b],
Johnny Lau, MD, MSc, FRCSC[b,*]

KEYWORDS

- Tendon transfers • Flexible forefoot deformities • Hammer toes • Hallux varus
- Angular toe deformities • Forefoot reconstruction

KEY POINTS

- Flexible forefoot deformities, such as hallux varus, clawed hallux, hammer toes, and angular lesser toe deformities, can be treated effectively with tendon transfers.
- Based on the presentation of the flexible forefoot deformities, tendon transfers can be used as the primary treatment or as adjuncts to bony procedures when there are components of fixed deformities.

Tendon transfers are powerful tools in the primary treatment of flexible forefoot deformities or as adjuncts to bony procedures. Deformities amenable to tendon transfer are hallux varus, clawed hallux, hammer toes, and angular lesser toe deformities.

GREAT TOE
Flexible Hallux Varus

Definition
Hallux varus has been noted as a complication of hallux valgus surgery with a reported incidence of 2% to 17%.[1–3] McBride first noted this deformity in 5.1% of patients treated with medial eminence removal, medial capsulorrhaphy, and fibular sesmoidectomy.[4] Hallux varus does not cause significant complaints unless the deformity is greater than 10° to 15°, primarily due to the resultant cosmetic appearance, or pain due to first metatarsophalangeal (MTP) degeneration or rubbing of the distal phalanx medially.[5] Hallux varus has been classified as either static or dynamic, and uniplanar and multiplanar, respectively.[6–9]

Static hallux varus is a flexible, passively correctable entity.[5] Most of the deformity occurs at the first MTP joint in the frontal plane. The deformity is commonly the result of excessive excision of the medial eminence, with the bunionectomy initiated lateral to the sagittal groove.[2]

[a] Division of Orthopaedics, Department of Surgery, University of Toronto, University Health Network-Toronto Western Division, 399 Bathurst Street 1 East 427, Toronto, Ontario M5T 2S8, Canada; [b] University Health Network-Toronto Western Division, 399 Bathurst Street, 1 East 438, Toronto, Ontario M5T 2S8, Canada
* Corresponding author.
E-mail address: drjohnnylau@gmail.com

Foot Ankle Clin N Am 19 (2014) 123–137
http://dx.doi.org/10.1016/j.fcl.2013.11.003
1083-7515/14/$ – see front matter © 2014 Elsevier Inc. All rights reserved.

Flexible deformities have been corrected by a variety of techniques, including the abductor hallucis, extensor digitorum brevis tendon, and the extensor hallucis longus (EHL) tendon[6,10,11] transfer.

Physical examination

A uniplanar hallux varus deformity is easily noted on examination. On assessment of the deformity, the deformity is passively correctable to neutral without much difficulty. The first MTP is then taken through a range of motion in the corrected position to ensure that there is no pain in the midrange of motion that could be the result of joint degeneration. Extent of joint degeneration can be confirmed on standing radiographs of the foot. In addition, passive correctability of the toe can be illustrated radiographically by taping the great toe in a corrected position and obtaining an anteroposterior standing radiography to confirm this reduction visually.

Split transfer of the EHL tendon in flexible hallux varus deformity

This procedure can be done for flexible hallux varus deformity without any osseous deformity.[12] It is best reserved for patients complaining of painful calluses along the distal phalanx with increasing varus alignment. First MTP degeneration is a contraindication to this reconstructive procedure.

A medial release is first done through a medial incision over the MTP. The capsule is defined and the dorsal medial hallucal nerve is protected. A VY lengthening of the capsule is then performed. A dorsal curvilinear incision is made with the start point just lateral to the insertion of the EHL and carried laterally toward the interval between the first and second metatarsals in the first web space. This incision is then carried medially to end at the lateral border of the EHL at the first metatarso-cuneiform joint. The EHL is split in line with its fibers. The distal lateral portion of the split is detached off of the distal phalanx and transferred under the intermetatarsal ligament of the first and second metatarsal from proximal to distal, after the end is whip-stitched with a nonabsorbable suture. The ligament acts as a pulley, allowing the EHL tendon transfer to pull the hallux plantar and lateral to the axis of the first MTP joint. A 4.0-mm drill is then used to make a tunnel from dorsomedial to plantar lateral in the proximal phalanx 1.5 cm proximal to the first MTP joint. The tendon is then passed from lateral to medial in this tunnel and secured with an interference screw or sutured to itself (**Fig. 1**). Another option is a suture anchor placed laterally in the proximal phalanx versus transosseous.[13,14]

Outcomes and complications

Fuhrmann[14] noted a decrease in range of motion of the first MTP joint in 7 of 12 patients. This decreased range of motion is likely due to the tenodesis effect of the tendon transfer. Alignment is generally improved with minimal residual varus that is not clinically evident in most cases and ground contract is improved. Fuhrmann[14] noted that 5 of 12 patients had an average varus position of 14° on radiographs, but only 2 of these 5 noted it clinically.

Endobutton technique for flexible hallux varus deformity

Although there are no long-term results, the endobutton procedure offers an alternative to the EHL tendon transfer.

A medial incision is made over the first MTP and the capsule is released vertically in line with and 1 cm proximal to the first MTP. At this point, if the first proximal phalanx continues to be deviated medially at the first MTP, the abductor hallucis tendon can be released from the base of the proximal phalanx. A second incision is made over the first web space, adjacent to the first MTP. The lateral capsule is incised and a vertical

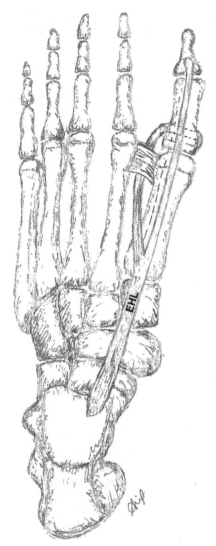

Fig. 1. The tendon is passed from lateral to medial in this tunnel and secured with an interference screw or sutured to itself.

capsulotomy is created for future plication in a pants-over-vest fashion once the hallux varus deformity is corrected. A guide wire for the mini-tightrope device is placed from distal medial in the proximal aspect of the proximal first phalanx (1 cm distal to the first MTP joint) to proximal lateral in the proximal aspect of the proximal phalanx (5 mm distal to the first MTP joint). This pin is overdrilled with a cannulated drill. The proximal limb of the endobutton is passed through this proximal phalanx drill hole from medial to lateral. A similar technique is used in the distal first metatarsal with the tunnel positioned 1 to 2 cm proximal to the first MTP on the medial aspect and 5 mm proximal in the lateral aspect. At this point the proximal limb of the endobutton is passed across the lateral aspect of the first MTP and through the distal first metatarsal tunnel from lateral to medial. In the lateral view, the metatarsal tunnel is just dorsal to the longitudinal axis and just plantar to the longitudinal axis in the proximal phalanx. The first MTP joint is then reduced and confirmed fluoroscopically, and the endobutton is tightened down. The lateral capsule is then plicated in a pants-over-vest fashion.

CLAWED HALLUX
Definition

Clawed hallux is a deformity of the great toe in which flexion of the first interphalangeal joint (IP) and extension of the first MTP joint occurs.[15] The deformity is a result of imbalance between the extrinsic muscles of the first ray, which include peroneus longus, EHL, and flexor hallucis longus (FHL).[15] This imbalance can be seen in pes cavovarus, where there is an imbalance between the tibialis anterior and the peroneus longus. In addition to the extrinsics, there can be weakness of the intrinsics and plantar fascial contractures.

Physical examination
The patient presents with pain and callusing under the first metatarsal head and overlying the dorsal IP joint. The IP joint is passively correctable and improves with plantar flexion of the ankle.

Surgical treatment of flexible claw toe deformity
The following 2 procedures can be used to correct a flexible claw toe deformity with flexion of the first IP joint and extension of the first MTP joint. A modified Jones procedure can be used in pathologic abnormalities such as Charcot-Marie-Tooth disease. However, when there is concern for the development of first MTP stiffness, an FHL transfer can be used to preserve function of the EHL and motion of the IP joint.

The modified Jones procedure
The great toe IP joint is approached with a transverse incision.[16–21] An arthrotomy of the IP joint is made and collaterals are released. The IP joint is prepared for fusion using standard techniques. The EHL tendon is identified and tagged with a 2.0 nonabsorbable suture and then released off the distal phalanx, before the preparation of the IP joint. The IP fusion is secured with a 4.0-mm cannulated screw or other construct of the surgeon's choice. A dorsal midline incision is made over the distal first metatarsal overlying the head-neck junction. The previously tagged EHL is delivered into the proximal wound. A 4.0 drill bit is used to make a drill hole in the metatarsal neck from medial to lateral. The EHL tendon is then passed from medial to lateral and sutured back to itself, with the ankle in neutral dorsiflexion and the deformity corrected (**Fig. 2**).

Flexor hallucis longus tendon transfer to proximal phalanx
Outcomes of the modified Jones, in regards to the lack of dorsiflexion and the stiff great toe, has led to the development of an alternative transfer of the FHL tendon from the first distal phalanx to the base of the proximal phalanx.[22,23] It has been suggested that the FHL transfer procedure preserves the function of the EHL and does not require fusion of the IP joint.[22]

A medial incision is made along the hallux overlying the proximal phalanx just distal to the IP joint and extended to the distal first metatarsal. Blunt dissection is used to avoid the plantar medial neurovascular bundle, staying on the bone. The FHL tendon is identified and the sheath is incised in line with its fibers. The FHL is tagged distally with a 2.0 nonabsorbable suture and then released from its insertion on the distal phalanx. The metaphyseal-diaphyseal junction is then identified dorsally, and a 4.0-mm drill is used to make a drill hole from dorsal to plantar in the proximal first phalanx. The FHL tendon is then passed from plantar to dorsal through the tunnel and wrapped

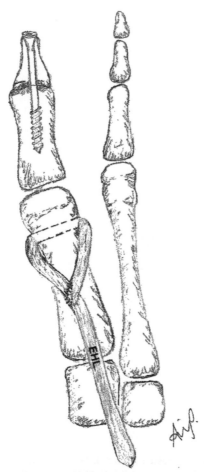

Fig. 2. The EHL tendon is passed from medial to lateral and sutured back to itself, with the ankle in neutral dorsiflexion and the deformity corrected.

medially over the proximal phalanx. It is then secured to itself and the local periosteum or secured with an interference screw (**Fig. 3**).

Flexor hallucis longus tendon transfer to EHL tendon transfer: a minimally invasive approach

A 1-cm longitudinal incision is made on the plantar aspect of the proximal aspect of the proximal phalanx.[24] The FHL is identified and its sheath is incised. The FHL is tagged with a 2.0-mm nonabsorbable suture and the tendon is released off the distal phalanx. Another longitudinal incision is made dorsally over the proximal phalanx. A 4.0-mm drill bit is used to make a tunnel from dorso-distal to plantar-proximal. The FHL tendon is then transferred from plantar to dorsal and sutured to the extensor hallucis tendon with the deformity corrected.

Outcomes and Complications

Both the Jones and the FHL transfers were equally effective in correcting deformities at the MTP and IP joints with the benefit of avoiding IP fusion with the FHL transfer, a considered benefit.[25]

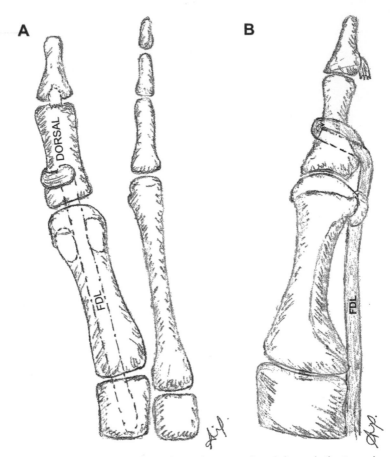

Fig. 3. (*A, B*) The FHL tendon is passed from plantar to dorsal through the tunnel and wrapped medially over the proximal phalanx. It is then secured to itself and the local periosteum or secured with an interference screw.

The modified Jones procedure

Catching of the great toe has been noted after this procedure.[21] However, even if patients reported catching, they were either "very pleased" or "pleased with reservations."[25] Recurrence of the claw toe deformity has been reported and attributed to the regeneration of the distal EHL stump.[26] In addition, stiffness of the great toe can be considered a downside of this procedure.[22]

Flexor hallucis longus tendon transfer to proximal phalanx

Flexor hallucis longus tendon transfer to proximal phalanx is an acceptable treatment in regards to deformity correction in hallux claw toe deformity with pain relief and patient satisfaction.[23] Alignment appears to be maintained on follow-up; however, return to strenuous activity may be limited.[23]

Flexor hallucis longus tendon transfer to EHL tendon transfer: a minimally invasive approach

The claw toe deformity was corrected in 7 of 7 patients.[24]

LESSER TOES
Flexible Hammer Toes

Definition
A hammer toe deformity is focused at the proximal IP joint of the lesser toes. The middle phalanx is flexed in relation to the proximal phalanx and the MTP joint is often hyperextended.[27] The relationship of the distal IP joint can be variable with reports of flexion, neutral, and extension posturing.[28,29] The patients generally present with pain due to pressure over the dorsal proximal IP joint, causing constraining foot wear issues.

These deformities are a result of disruption of the balance between static stabilizers, such as the plantar plate and ligaments, and dynamic stabilizers, such as the intrinsics and extrinics. Weakness of the intrinsics allows the first MTP joint to extend, which results in the long flexor tendons flexing the PIP joint. In addition, plantar plate laxity may lead to MTP joint hyperextension and nonphysiologic PIP joint flexion.[30]

Physical examination
In general, there is flexion of the proximal interphalangeal joint (PIP) with variable degrees of distal interphalangeal joint (DIP) flexion and MTP joint extension on examination. It is important to assess the flexibility of the PIP joint and define it as either flexible or fixed. In addition, it is important to assess the MTP joint for a hyperextension deformity (a complex hammer toe deformity) because this may need to be realigned in the same setting as the PIP.[27] In regards to the PIP joint, if the deformity is passively correctable, it is considered to be flexible. To assess the tightness of the flexor tendons, the ankle should be moved through an arc of dorsiflexion to plantar flexion.[27] If the PIP joint corrects to neutral as the ankle is brought into plantar flexion, this is a flexible hammer toe deformity and a flexible hammer toe deformity is the result of a flexor digitorum longus (FDL) tendon contracture.[28]

Surgical treatment of flexible hammer toe deformity
Flexor to extensor tendon transfer The flexor to extensor transfer allows the FDL to act as an intrinsic on the proximal phalanx, allowing for its depression, and at the same time avoids its native deforming force on the distal phalanx.[31,32]

A longitudinal incision is made just distal to the proximal plantar flexion crease. Soft tissue is retracted and the FDL sheath is identified and split longitudinally. The longitudinal incision helps avoid damage to the adjacent neurovascular structures.[33] A mosquito curved clamp is used to identify the tendon and place it under tension and split longitudinally (**Fig. 4**). The distal ends of the tendon are tagged with nonabsorbable suture on a noncutting needle. Distally, the FDL tendon is released from the base of the distal phalanx. A longitudinal incision is made over the midportion of the proximal phalanx. A curved mosquito clamp is passed from dorsal to plantar on both the medial and the lateral aspects of the proximal phalanx, staying close to bone and above the extensor hood to protect the neurovascular digital bundles. The 2 aspects of the split FDL tendon are then passed on either side of the proximal phalanx using these mosquito clamps and then tied over the extension expansion and to itself with the nonabsorbable suture (**Fig. 5**). The FDL tendon transfer is sutured with the toe held in approximately 20° of plantar flexion.[27] A K-wire is used to stabilize the construct by pinning from the distal phalanx to the proximal phalanx. This pin is removed in approximately 2 to 6 weeks.

Flexor to extensor tendon transfer Instead of splitting the FDL in a plantar fashion and passing it around the proximal phalanx, the tendon can be harvested in similar fashion, as a single unit, and passed from plantar to dorsal through a drill hole in the junction of

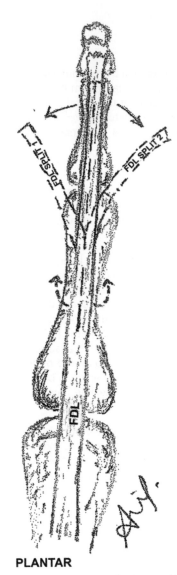

PLANTAR

Fig. 4. A mosquito curved clamp is used to identify the tendon and place it under tension and split longitudinally.

the middle and distal third of the proximal phalanx.[34,35] A 2.0- to 2.5-mm drill bit can be used. Before making the drill hole, dissection dorsally needs to be carried down to the extensor sheath, which is then split in line with the incision and can be sutured to the extensor hood with a 3.0 to 2.0 nonabsorbable suture on a noncutting needle, or with a 4.0 absorbable suture.

Outcomes and Complications

Potential complications are transient swelling and numbness, which tend to subside over time.[27,28] Other potential sources of complication are related to the K-wire. K-wires may need to be removed if there is any concern of postoperative vascular insufficiency,

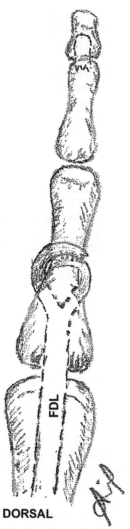

DORSAL

Fig. 5. The 2 aspects of the split FDL tendon are then passed on either side of the proximal phalanx using these mosquito clamps and then tied over the extension expansion and to itself with the nonabsorbable suture.

which is rare. Treatment of vascular insufficiency, before pulling the pin, should be warming of the toe with warm saline, and then adjusting the K-wire. Lidocaine around the neurovascular bundle can help with smooth muscle relaxation as can nitro paste.[35]

After a flexor to extensor transfer, patients loose the ability to actively flex their DIP joints and therefore curl their toes. They can retain passive but not active function of the IP joints, and over time they can develop PIP stiffness.[27] PIP stiffness has been reported in 60% of cases and is one of the main reasons for dissatisfaction in this procedure.[36] Although flexor to extensor tendon transfer achieves MTP joint congruity and reliably improves pain due to instability, postoperative mobilization appears to be the key to diminishing postoperative stiffness, with removal of pins advised earliest at 2 weeks.[37] As such, it is always prudent to discuss with patients that they will trade an unstable deformity for a stiff toe with minimal function.

An 89% satisfaction rate was reported by Boyer and DeOrio[33] in fixed and flexible hammer toes. Previous literature has shown satisfaction rates of 89% to 95%. Thompson and Deland[37] found that all of their patients had some amount of pain relief with 8 of 13 being completely pain-free.

There is an approximately 20% chance of recurrence of the deformity.[35] This recurrence is likely the result preoperative stiffness and/or preoperative MTP extension, which was not adequately evaluated and addressed intraoperatively with more extensive soft tissue releases with or without bone shortening procedures. Recurrence is also due to inadequate tensioning and positioning of the transfer.

LESSER TOE ANGULAR DEFORMITIES
Definition

Crossover toe deformity and isolated MTP joint angular deformity can result in significant pain because of pressure effects on adjacent toes and from shoe wear. These deformities can result from intrinsic and extrinsic causes, such as trauma, inflammatory arthritis, congenital deformities, and constraining footwear.[30] Isolated MTP deformity is seen as a valgus or varus angulation at the MTP joint and is often associated with great toe angular deformity. A crossover second toe deformity is defined by the second toe crossing dorsally over the first.

Angular coronal plane deformities can result from a cascade of trauma or synovitis, followed by subluxation and dorsal or inferiomedial dislocation of the proximal phalanges on the metatarsal heads. Other findings are laxity of the collateral ligaments, which provide stability in the transverse plane and resist dorsal subluxation of the proximal phalanx on the metatarsal head. The medial collateral (MCL) and lateral collateral ligaments (LCL) originate from the dorsal metatarsal heads and insert distally plantar on the plantar plate and base of the proximal phalanx. Imbalance between intrinsics and extrinsics can result in lesser toe deformities, because the intrinsics in their normal anatomic relationship act as MTP flexors and PIP and DIP extensors. In the case of the second crossover toe, there is laxity and subsequent rupture of the LCL and lateral capsule. In addition, a long second metatarsal is associated with attenuation of the first dorsal interosseous tendon and plantar plate.

Physical Examination

In second toe crossover deformity, the patient presents with a dorsomedially subluxed second toe, which is overlying the first toe. There can be hyperextension and varus angulation at the MTP and hyperflexion of the PIP joint. There can be pain and callusing over the dorsal PIP and plantar metatarsal head with rubbing between the 2 toes. There may be instability of the plantar plate, which is identified with the drawer test. The deformity at the MTP is passively correctable as is the PIP flexion.

Isolated coronal angular deformities of the MTP joints are passively correctable and have pain where there is pressure between the toes.

As in hammer toe deformities, the flexibility of the PIP joint needs to be assessed and defined as either flexible or fixed. In addition, it is important to assess the MTP joint for a hyperextension deformity (a complex hammer toe deformity) as this may need to be realigned in the same setting as the PIP through bony fusion of the PIP and possible Weil osteotomy of the distal metatarsal.[27]

Surgical Treatment of Flexible Lesser Angular Toe Deformities

In the setting of dynamic or fixed PIP hammer toe deformities, these deformities should be addressed with separate techniques, as should MTP hyperextension and plantar plate disruption. Correction of the flexible first MTP angular deformities, which could be fixed in isolation or in conjunction with PIP and MTP sagittal deformities, is discussed.

MCL and medial capsule contracture in association with LCL and lateral capsule attenuation/disruption can be treated with soft tissue balancing techniques, including releasing the contracted MCL off the metatarsal head and phalanx from dorsal to plantar, and repairing the attenuated LCL in a shortened position.[30] This shortening can then be stabilized with a K-wire, which is removed in 6 weeks.

Tendon transfer techniques can also be used to further dynamically stabilize the coronal deformities.

As mentioned in the physical examination section, fixed components of PIP flexion deformities may need to be addressed with bony PIP fusion and MTP extension deformities may need to be addressed with MTP decompression and possible bony work in the form of Weil distal metatarsal osteotomies.

Extensor digitorum brevis transfer

A dorsal incision is made over the proximal phalanx and distal metatarsal of the affected digit.[30] The extensor digitorum brevis tendon (EDB) is identified and followed proximally. The MTP joint capsule is entered transversely and the contracted collateral ligament, usually the MCL, is released off of the metatarsal head and phalanx from dorsal to plantar. The extensor digitorum longus tendon (EDL) is then identified and followed proximally. The EDL is then z-lengthened and both its ends are tagged with nonabsorbable 3.0- to 2.0-mm sutures. Four centimeters proximal to the MTP joint, the EDB is secured with two 3.0- to 2.0-mm nonabsorbable sutures, and the tendon is transected between the 2 sutures. The distal EDB tendon is then passed from distal to proximal under the transverse intermetatarsal ligament on the convex side of the MTP coronal deformity (**Fig. 6**). The EDB is then appropriately tensioned and secured to its proximal stump, with the coronal MTP deformity congruently corrected and secured with a K-wire from distal phalanx to distal metatarsal. The K-wire is pulled at 6 weeks.

Modified extensor digitorum tendon transfer

A dorsal incision is made over the proximal phalanx and distal metatarsal of the affected digit.[30] The EDL tendon is identified and followed proximally. The EDL is then z-lengthened and both its ends are tagged with nonabsorbable 3.0- to 2.0-mm sutures. The extensor EDB is then identified and followed proximally. The MTP joint capsule is entered transversely and the contracted collateral ligament, usually the MCL, is released off the metatarsal head and phalanx from dorsal to plantar. Four centimeters proximal to the MTP joint, the EDB is secured with two 3.0- to 2.0-mm nonabsorbable sutures, and the tendon is transected between the 2 sutures. An oblique bone tunnel is made in the proximal aspect of the proximal phalanx using a 2.5-mm drill bit and is oriented distal in the proximal phalanx to the convex side of the deformity, which is generally proximal-lateral in the proximal phalanx. The distal stump of the EDL is passed through the bone tunnel from medial to lateral, or from the concave side of the deformity to the convex side of the deformity. This EDL tendon is then passed from distal to proximal under the transverse intermetatarsal ligament on the convex side of the MTP deformity (**Fig. 7**). The transferred distal stump of the EDL tendon is then tensioned and secured side-to-side with the proximal stump of the EDB, with the coronal MTP deformity congruently corrected and secured with a K-wire from distal phalanx to distal metatarsal. The proximal stump of the EDL is then sutured to the distal stump of the EDB. The K-wire is pulled at 6 weeks.

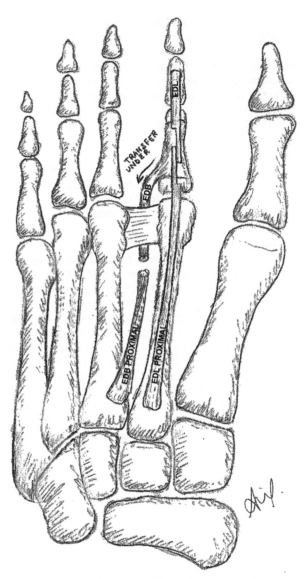

Fig. 6. The distal EDB tendon is then passed from distal to proximal under the transverse intermetatarsal ligament on the convex side of the MTP coronal deformity.

Outcomes and Complications

Complications include inability to obtain anatomic correction of the deformity, and recurrence of crossover deformity.[30]

Haddad and colleagues[38] showed that 24 of 31 patients were satisfied with their surgical correction from either the EDB or the flexor-extensor tendon transfers. Although there was no statistical significance between FDL and EDB tendon transfer, the authors thought that EDB transfer resulted in better mobility and range of motion of the toe and subsequent improved satisfaction, better pain control, and diminished recurrence of deformity, as compared with FDL transfer.[38]

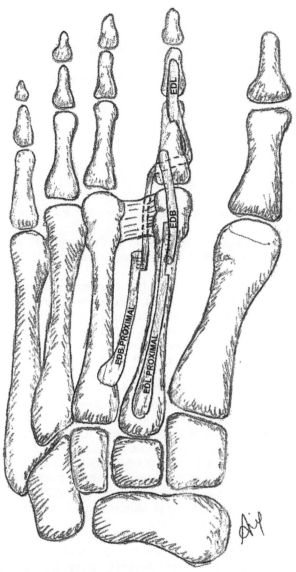

Fig. 7. The distal stump of the EDL is passed through the bone tunnel from medial to lateral, or from the concave side of the deformity to the convex side of the deformity. This EDL tendon is then passed from distal to proximal under the transverse intermetatarsal ligament on the convex side of the MTP deformity.

SUMMARY

Flexible forefoot deformities, such as hallux varus, clawed hallux, hammer toes, and angular lesser toe deformities, can be treated effectively with tendon transfers. Based on the presentation of the flexible forefoot deformities, tendon transfers can be used as the primary treatment or as adjuncts to bony procedures when there are components of fixed deformities.

REFERENCES

1. Peterson DA, Zilberfarb JL, Greene MA, et al. Avascular necrosis of the first meta-tarsal head: incidence in distal osteotomy combined with lateral soft tissue release. Foot Ankle Int 1994;15:59–63.
2. Trnka HJ, Zettl R, Hungford M, et al. Acquired hallux varus and clinical tolerability. Foot Ankle Int 1997;18:593–7.
3. Miller JW. Acquired hallux varus: a preventable and correctable disorder. J Bone Joint Surg Am 1975;57:183–8.
4. McBride ED. The conservative operation for "bunions": end results and refine-ments of technique. JAMA 1935;105:1164–8.
5. Mann RA, Coughlin MJ. Adult hallux valgus. In: Mann RA, Coughlin MJ, editors. Surgery of the foot and ankle. 6th edition. St Louis (MO): Mosby-Year Book; 1993. p. 167–296.
6. Hawkins F. Acquired hallux varus: cause, prevention, and correction. Clin Orthop 1971;76:169–76.
7. Richardson EG. Disorders of the hallux. In: Crenshaw AH, editor. Campbell's operative orthopaedics, vol. 4, 8th edition. St Louis (MO): Mosby-Year Book; 1992. p. 2615–92.
8. Juliano PJ, Myerson MS, Cunningham BW. Biomechanical assessment of a new tenodesis for correction of hallux varus. Foot Ankle Int 1996;17:17–20.
9. Myerson MS, Komenada GA. Results of hallux varus correction using an extensor hillocks brevis tenodesis. Foot Ankle Int 1996;17:21–7.
10. Johnson KA. Dissatisfaction following hallux valgus surgery. Surgery of the foot and ankle. New York: Raven Press; 1989. p. 35–68.
11. Johnson KA, Spiegl PV. Extensor hallucis longus transfer for hallux varus defor-mity. J Bone Joint Surg Am 1984;66(5):681–6.
12. Lau JT, Myerson M. Modified split extensor hallucis longus tendon transfer for correction of hallux varus. Foot Ankle Int 2002;23(12):1138–40.
13. Mann RA. Hallux varus: split extensor hallux longus transfer. In: Wülker N, Stephens MM, Cracchiolo A III, editors. An atlas of foot and ankle surgery. London, New York: Taylor & Francis; 2005. p. 45–8.
14. Fuhrmann R. Split transfer of the extensor hallucis longus tendon on flexible hallux varus deformity. Oper Orthop Traumatol 2008;20(3):274–82.
15. Olson SL, Ledoux WR, Ching RP, et al. Muscular imbalances resulting in a clawed hallux. Foot Ankle Int 2003;24:477–85.
16. Barnett M, Manoli A, Sangeorzan BJ, et al. Comprehensive correction of cavova-rus foot deformity. In: Wiesel SW, editor. Operative techniques in orthopaedic sur-gery, vol. 4. Philadelphia: Wolters Kluwer/Lippincott Williams & Wilkins; 2011. p. 3889–90 Chapter 55.
17. Tynan MC, Klenerman L. The modified Robert Jones tendon transfer in cases of pes cavus and clawed hallux. Foot Ankle Int 1994;15(2):68–71.
18. Giannini S, Girolami M, Ceccarelli F, et al. Modified Jones operation in the treat-ment of pes cavovarus. Ital J Orthop Traumatol 1985;11(2):165–70.
19. de Palma L, Colonna E, Travasi M. The modified Jones procedure for pes cavo-varus with claw hallux. J Foot Ankle Surg 1997;36(4):279–83.
20. Jones R. The soldier's foot and the treatment of common deformities of the foot. Br Med J 1916;1:749–52.
21. Breusch SJ, Wenz W, Doderlein L. Function after correction of a clawed great toe by a modified Robert Jones transfer. J Bone Joint Surg Br 2000;82: 250–4.

22. Hansen ST. Functional reconstruction of the foot and ankle. Philadelphia: Lippincott Williams & Wilkins; 2000. p. 453.
23. Steensma MR, Jabara M, Anderson JG, et al. Flexor hallucis longus tendon transfer for hallux claw toe deformity and vertical instability of the metatarsophalangeal joint. Foot Ankle Int 2006;27(9):689–92.
24. Lui TH. Flexor hallucis longus tendon to extensor hallucis longus tendon transfer for flexible hallux claw toe deformity: a minimally invasive approach. Foot Ankle Int 2013;34(2):303–6.
25. Elias FN, Yuen TJ, Olson SL, et al. Correction of clawed hallux deformity: comparison of the Jones procedure and FHL transfer in a cadaver model. Foot Ankle Int 2007;28(3):369–76.
26. M'Bamali EI. Results of modified Robert Jones operation for clawed hallux. Br J Surg 1975;62:647–50.
27. Coughlin M. Lesser toe abnormalities. Instr Course Lect 2003;52:421–44.
28. Coughlin M, Mann R. Lesser toe deformities. In: Coughlin MJ, Mann RA, editors. Surgery of the foot and ankle. 7th edition. St Lois (MO): Mosby Yearbook; 1999. p. 320–91.
29. Coughlin MJ. Lesser toe deformities. Orthopedics 1987;10:63–75.
30. Flemister AS Jr, Giordano BD. Angular deformity of the lesser toes. In: Wiesel SW, editor. Operative techniques in orthopaedic surgery, vol. 4. Wolters Kluwer/Lippincott Williams & Wilkins; 2011. p. 3714–29 Chapter 34.
31. Barbari SG, Brevig K. Correction of clawtoes by the Girdlestone Taylor flexor-extensor transfer procedure. Foot Ankle 1984;5:67–73.
32. Kirschner J, Wagner E. Girdlestone-Taylor flexor-extensor tendon transfer. Tech Foot Ankle Surg 2004;3:91–9.
33. Boyer ML, DeOrio JK. Transfer of the flexor digitorum longus for the correction of lesser toe deformities. Foot Ankle 2007;28:422–30.
34. Kuwada GT. A retrospective analysis of modification of the flexor tendon transfer for correction of hammer toe. J Foot Surg 1988;27:57–9.
35. Wagner E. Flexor-to-extensor tendon transfer for flexible hammer toe deformity. In: Wiesel SW, editor. Operative techniques in orthopaedic surgery, vol. 4. Wolters Kluwer/Lippincott Williams & Wilkins; 2011. p. 3688–95 Chapter 31.
36. Cyphers SM, Feiwell E. Review of the Girdlestone-Taylopr procedure for clawtoes in myelodysplasia. Foot Ankle 1988;8:229–33.
37. Thompson FM, Deland JT. Flexor tendon transfer for metatarsophalangeal instability of the second toe. Foot Ankle 1993;14:385–8.
38. Haddad SL, Sabbah RC, Resch S, et al. Results of flexor-to-extensor and extensor brevis tendon transfers for correction of the crossover second toe deformity. Foot Ankle Int 1992;20:781–8.

Index

Note: Page numbers of article titles are in **boldface** type.

Foot Ankle Clin N Am 19 (2014) 139–164
http://dx.doi.org/10.1016/S1083-7515(14)00009-6
1083-7515/14/$ – see front matter © 2014 Elsevier Inc. All rights reserved.

Moving?

Make sure your subscription moves with you!

To notify us of your new address, find your **Clinics Account Number** (located on your mailing label above your name), and contact customer service at:

Email: journalscustomerservice-usa@elsevier.com

800-654-2452 (subscribers in the U.S. & Canada)
314-447-8871 (subscribers outside of the U.S. & Canada)

Fax number: 314-447-8029

Elsevier Health Sciences Division
Subscription Customer Service
3251 Riverport Lane
Maryland Heights, MO 63043

*To ensure uninterrupted delivery of your subscription, please notify us at least 4 weeks in advance of move.

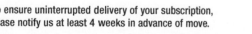

Printed and bound by CPI Group (UK) Ltd, Croydon, CR0 4YY

03/10/2024

01040496-0016